IT'S NOT
ABOUT
YOU,

EXCEPT
WHEN IT IS

A Field Manual for Parents
of Addicted Children

Barbara Victoria

CENTRAL RECOVERY PRESS, LAS VEGAS, NEVADA

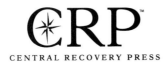

CENTRAL RECOVERY PRESS

Central Recovery Press (CRP) is committed to publishing exceptional materials addressing addiction treatment, recovery, and behavioral health care topics, including original and quality books, audio/visual communications, and web-based new media. Through a diverse selection of titles, we seek to contribute a broad range of unique resources for professionals, recovering individuals and their families, and the general public.

For more information, visit www.centralrecoverypress.com.

Central Recovery Press, Las Vegas, NV 89129

Publisher: Central Recovery Press
3321 N. Buffalo Drive
Las Vegas, NV 89129

17 16 15 14 13 12   1 2 3 4 5

ISBN-13: 978-1-936290-94-9 (paper)
ISBN-13: 978-1-937612-02-3 (e-book)

Author photo by Rogena Walden. Used with permission.

Publisher's Note: This book contains general information about addiction, codependency, and family relationships. Central Recovery Press makes no representations or warranties in relation to the information herein; it is not an alternative to medical advice from your doctor or other professional healthcare provider.

Our books represent the experiences and opinions of their authors only. Every effort has been made to ensure that events, institutions, and statistics presented in our books as facts are accurate and up-to-date. To protect their privacy, some of the names of people and institutions have been changed.

Cover design and illustrations by Marisa Jackson
Interior design and layout by Marisa Jackson

SPECIAL PRAISE FOR
It's Not About You, Except When It Is

"If you could distill all of the substance abuse texts written for professionals into one book that tells parents what they need to know, in a way they need to hear it, so they can use it, you would get this book. This is a compelling, heart-rending story of a mother earning wisdom, and her willingness to share that with others. I fully intend to use it as a resource and guide for families who come to me seeking help for their child (of any age) who is dealing with an addiction."

—Steve Humphries-Wadsworth, PhD, LMFT
CLINICAL DIRECTOR, YELLOWSTONE BEHAVIORAL HEALTH CENTER

"I know of no other book that provides so much assistance to every parent with children suffering from addiction. This beautifully written book was crafted from true life experience and an open heart.

Addiction is a thief both to the addicted child and the parent. This is a long-awaited book that offers promise and hope to the struggling parent and the total family. My gratitude to Barbara Victoria for the meaningful, purposeful, and compassionate gift she has given all parents and families who deal with the moment-by-moment trials and tribulations of an addicted child."

—Linda Tatum, LMFT

"Parents. Ignorance is NOT bliss when traveling with your child through drug and alcohol addiction. Barbara Victoria's manual offers the needed 'smarts' for the journey through this bleak landscape. Recover hope and retrain your thinking as you follow her voice out of the wilderness— reclaiming your sanity and your life."

—Deborah M. Smith, ACC
CERTIFIED LIFE COACH

IT'S NOT
ABOUT
YOU,

EXCEPT
WHEN IT IS

THESE WORDS ARE DEDICATED to my first support group, which originated as a group of parents seeking to bolster one another as our loved ones battled addiction or the two-headed dragon of mental illness and addiction. The group was never restricted to women, but it evolved through time into a core of mothers, led by one heaven-sent clinical social worker who brought us all together two Monday evenings a month for several years. All love to each of you!

To all mothers and fathers of children who are addicts. To all the siblings, aunts and uncles, and grandmothers and grandfathers who, by virtue of love, have suffered with a loved one's addiction. To all "blended" families; and specifically to my husband, William, who struggled to comprehend what we were going through and "walked the ridge" when I had to go it alone—which was often. To my loved one's father and his wife, who walk the walk. To my firstborn. To my siblings. To friends who have been more than friends.

To my loved one, through whom I entered this journey and learned to grow in incalculable ways of being and feeling and thinking and doing. *I love you every day and every night, beyond all days and nights.*

And always, to Victoria Barbara, who seems to have passed on a modicum of her extraordinary strength and perseverance to her daughter.

• TABLE OF CONTENTS •

• AUTHOR'S NOTE •

I use the terms "daughter/son," "daughter," and "son" interchangeably to represent each of our children who unwittingly set us on a formidable and extraordinary journey. May the purity of the primal love that exists between parent and child initiate in them a resolve to heal their lives and embrace all that we, their mothers and fathers, could ever want for them: the gift of being who they truly are.

• PROLOGUE •

SOMETIMES MY FATHER would call me "Princess" when I was a little girl, and I relished it. As the youngest in the family, with two older brothers, I often felt invisible. But calling me Princess pleased him, and being called Princess made me feel good. That's when I learned the value of pleasing and how to make it happen.

What I really loved, however, was when he called me "Bobby." A boy's name for a nickname put me closer to boy status. Boys did much more interesting things than girls when I was growing up in the mid-1940s and 1950s—going on expeditions in the woods and climbing trees and camping. My father and brothers would invite me along sometimes to go squirrel hunting, but my short legs would get entangled in underbrush as I struggled to keep up with them. Still, I persevered. That pleased my father, too.

I learned to cut my hair like Peter Pan—my "superhero," though there was no such term for such characters at that time.

I could climb to the tops of trees and play baseball on a real diamond with the big boys, but I could never be a real boy. Keeping up would be as good as it would get, so I valued being called Princess once in a while and making my father smile. This also secured my own niche in the family. Later in life I would have to rewire this behavior, but the attention felt good and offered more status than being "just a girl" in the 1950s.

Alcohol had no particular presence in our home. My father enjoyed a cold beer or a dry martini, and I remember my grandfather mixing manhattans for the grown-ups for family get-togethers, but drinking was mostly for special occasions.

I don't remember my mother drinking much at all. She may have had a rare glass of wine, but her prize decanter held colored water that she would change depending upon the holiday season. Tea was her beverage of choice, and there was always a teapot on the table at mealtime. There were no taboos about alcohol; it just wasn't significant.

I was in my early twenties and in college when I watched my date pull a bottle from under the front seat of the car, draw several swallows of whiskey, and chase it with a can of 7-Up resting on the console. I had never seen anyone do that before, but I figured that must be the way people did things in the Southeast, where we were both in college. We enjoyed a dinner together and a couple of drinks, and dated for the next year before we were married.

My husband and I came from different regions of the country, and that designated me an outsider when I married into a close, rural family. I adored my mother-in-law and father-in-law and their extended families. The art of pleasing that I learned as a little girl began to serve me well as I learned to fit into a family system and a community where generation after generation had grown up and succeeding generations followed.

When our children were babies we moved to the family farm, where they were the fourth generation to live. Right away I learned that visiting a farm and living and working on a farm were vastly different, and the adjustment was extremely challenging for me. The better I got along and went along, the better it worked for everyone, it seemed. My "pleasing" personality was an asset. My mother-in-law became my mentor, whether she realized it or not, and I admired her country sensibilities and natural class. We had great fun together, and she taught me everything I know about country cooking. My father-in-law and I would fish together and share books, and I relished his attention as I had my father's. He became a second father to me.

Our early years on the farm were sweet indeed, with three generations living on neighboring acreage in a nuclear unit that was wholly our own. Sometimes it seemed like the center of the universe, and for our children I know it was. As they grew older and went off to kindergarten and grade school, they would get off the bus at their grandparents' after school until my husband or I came in from our off-farm work and took them down to the old farmhouse.

Beer and whiskey were staples in our households, and alcohol was always a fixture for family occasions. My mother-in-law and I would enjoy a drink together; I learned to love a cold beer or a 7 and 7, but like my father I seemed to have a physical limit.

Consumption for the men could be a beer or two by midmorning on a weekend, and in the evenings two or three beers with two or three shots of whiskey. There was always beer in the fridge and whiskey in the pantry. This didn't seem unusual to me; it's just the way it was and, for all I knew, always had been.

I cannot say when our youngest child first sampled alcohol. It could have been any time between elementary school and high school; liquor was always on hand and easy to access. Officially, however, I would say the beginning of a serious relationship with alcohol began in our child's late teens or early twenties, when mishaps and fender benders began to accumulate.

The real slide into addiction probably began with the first DUI at age nineteen. As a mother I was bereft, and the questions began: *What did we miss? What could or should we have done differently? What can we do better? How do we fix this?*

Beneath mounting uncertainties about what was happening to our teenager was the knowledge that the innocence that is the birthright of every child had been shattered. There was no way to bring it back or restore the pristine world that our child had known. Moreover, I sensed that this accident held far more import than a night in jail, fines, and DUI counseling. Something much deeper than youthful transgression had rent our family. After a few more years of transgressions and consequences and moving in and out of college, a pattern had emerged.

Another DUI may have gone down by the time my car was totaled—you think you will never forget the searing details of your child's life unraveling—and that was when I made a list of all the accidents and mishaps since high school. I offered the list to my husband and youngest offspring as a matter of concern and—I hoped—to get their attention. I noted that five of eight incidents were known to have been alcohol-related. To my utter dismay, I was roundly dismissed. Moreover, they agreed that I was being an alarmist. That was the end of it. After our "talk," which didn't turn out to be very long, it was clear to me that I was on the outside looking in at this evolving situation. Moreover, I was totally on my own.

Had I understood anything of how alcohol and other drugs can work physically on some people and not others, and how coping behaviors can morph those around them, I would have sought help for myself and discovered twelve-step recovery twenty years before I did. I was doing everything I knew how to do, but I simply didn't know enough. In the intervening years, I made a lot of mistakes. In fact, I became a poster child for codependence before I'd heard the word or understood the dynamic. I probably did just about everything wrong that a person can do. When I wasn't isolating myself, I was trying to help or manage everyone and everything around me except the person who needed help and managing the most, and that was me.

I was resolved that our now-adult child could be rescued. If my husband and I couldn't see eye-to-eye on what was happening, at least we were together in doing the "right" thing as parents. We were compassionate and understanding; we tried to meet every transgression with equanimity. We fixed, we fudged, and we were determined to get our child "over the hump." We stayed focused on the big picture.

We could right this wrong—we would. Life as we had all known it would resume. YES!

Throughout those years, I had no idea how our firstborn was impacted by the attention being focused on the welfare of our youngest. We were stumbling in the dark, not looking at the problem together when there was any clarity, and wholly ignorant of addiction. Our reflex was to rush to the child in need, and, given our limitations, I don't see how we could have done it any differently. We were operating on instinct when we needed smarts.

As the addictive behavior of our youngest child progressed year after year, neither of us saw the toll it was taking on our firstborn—the one who had been dotting all the I's and crossing all the T's was sidelined by crisis after crisis created by the addiction of the youngest child. If I could do this part of my life over I would pay better attention to what was going right with our firstborn, show more support, give more praise. Share the love we had. Instead, I allowed myself to be overtaken by fear and anxiety as I focused on the child in crisis. It doesn't matter that I didn't know any better. I was sending a false message to my firstborn: you are not as important. Insult was added to injury.

I also mishandled the differences with my husband and me. I felt dismissed by his inability to see or try to understand what was happening to our youngest child under our noses. It was obvious to me that something wasn't right. As my feelings morphed from anger to depression, the gulf between us widened. We couldn't come to terms with the circumstances of our offspring, let alone our marriage, which was being traumatized in many other ways.

I sought counseling for three stretches over a six-year period to work on my "baggage," which I knew to be considerable, but I could not communicate to my spouse the necessity of going together to address the problems that were ours. As I paid attention to my side of the road, I began to gain a different perspective. I gained tools that worked, and began to find a way out of the engulfing darkness. The distance between my husband and me continued to grow.

Within one year, my children lost three grandparents. My husband and I separated. For most of the next decade our youngest child slid further into addiction and into one crisis after another. The cycles of codependency came and went as we bumped along an uneasy bottom. Looking back at those years, I cannot believe that it went on as long as it did.

Several years passed, and my adult child earned a couple more DUIs. By then my husband and I had divorced, and I'd moved to another state where I married again. I had been working for a mental health agency for several years after seeking advice there to understand what was going on with my youngest child's addiction and depression. They offered me a position as a respite case manager, then as a mental health technician in a group home.

The clients I worked with were mentally ill and dual- or multiple-diagnosis patients managing mental illness and/or substance abuse (any of which could be plural). I became familiar with all the agencies and social services in our small town, the terminology they used, and how they worked and interacted.

You help someone to help himself or herself, right? My many ducks were in a row, and with the help of my former husband I brought our careening offspring to live with my husband and me while I began putting the grand plan into place. I thought that I knew exactly what to do and how to go about it. While I had learned by then that I could not *cure* addictive behavior, I knew how and where to direct someone who needed help.

Tapping into all the social service agencies that could be called upon entailed layers of paperwork and time to process, so through friends I lined up work that provided a place to live and a decent wage until my adult child was cleared to enter a twenty-eight-day treatment program.

And more wonderfulness was in store. A nearby community college was auctioning dormitory furniture to be replaced at the beginning of the fall term. For a mere $63 I was able to buy twin beds and mattresses, a dining table and four chairs, a sofa and two chairs for a living area, and a coffee table. It was decent furniture, and a start toward independent living one day.

The ducks were lining up right, and they were rockin' and rollin'! I put all the furniture into a storage locker while the necessary paperwork churned through the system to secure a place for my loved one in a twenty-eight-day treatment program near our home. With my residency and the documentation required for the program, we were able to have the treatment paid for by the state.

At the end of the twenty-eight days, I attended Family Day—actually two and a half days of workshops with parents alone, and parents together with their family members in treatment. What an eye-opener that was. I marveled at the diversity of parents, the span of our ages and backgrounds and histories. There were adults and teenagers in the program with all manner of addictions and behaviors.

Some of our sessions were strictly informative. I learned that alcohol is processed differently in the system of someone who can become addicted than in the system of someone who can drink without becoming addicted. This difference is systemic, an allergic reaction that has a genetic component.

I was amazed to hear that it is not how much a person drinks or the time of day that they consume that signifies alcoholic behavior, but *why* they drink and *how* alcohol affects them. I asked if chasing a juice glass of whiskey with a beer at nine o'clock in the morning was alcoholic behavior. The workshop leader said it was the relationship of the person to the substance (whether alcohol or other drugs, or a behavior) that determined whether he or she had addiction. Why a person uses a substance and how he or she is affected by it is the determining factor indicating addiction. A profound change in personality or behavior is significant, as is frequency of use. Click.

The discussion of the family dynamics that evolve to cope with addiction got my attention as well. The workshop leader described the shutting down of communication, the inability to discuss what was happening, reference at best to "a problem," the isolation among family members, and codependent coping behaviors such as tiptoeing, deferring, placating, and rescuing. *HELLO!*

Lights were switching on inside my head. The presenter was describing behaviors that were all too familiar in the family and extended family I had known. No labels were necessary. The use of alcohol had impacted several generations. Period. In the years I'd been learning how to be a farm wife, it seems I had also perfected the adaptive behaviors of a model codependent! I was utterly stunned.

Then I was angry. I had done the best I knew how to do at the time, but I hadn't known enough about what was impacting our family to affect change. It takes two to make or break a marriage, and I accepted my part in the separation, but I felt I had taken most of the responsibility for what was out in the open. Plenty had never been acknowledged, let alone discussed.

Then I was sad. An unspoken condition had wrapped around us all and ran through us. No one could possibly look at it directly, let alone identify it or do anything to change something that hadn't been recognized. In silence and in denial, none of us had a chance.

I also learned that addiction is a progressive disease that is manifest in people of all shapes and sizes and from all walks of life.

The workshop leader flatly refuted the term *functional alcoholic*. There is no such animal, he said. He described addiction to alcohol as an allergic reaction that affects people in as many different ways as there are addicts.

> **I also learned that addiction is a progressive disease that is manifest in people of all shapes and sizes and from all walks of life.**

Some addicts pass out in a gutter; some are confined to hospitals; some are in treatment programs; and some go to work and have families and live in nice homes and have money in the bank. Since my family's addiction problems centered on alcohol, I paid close attention to everything the counselors said pertaining to alcoholism; however, I also learned that the same things are true for all manifestations of addiction. There is no "prototype" for addiction, only the way the physical body processes substances.

After Family Day, I felt tender love and respect for my youngest child, who had been through so much for too many years, and regret that almost no one in the family understood. My adult child not was not an invisible user. Mostly it was revealed by court appearances reported in the local paper, which were hard to ignore. There was plenty of talk among plenty of people who had opinions based on what they saw. What they knew was far less.

Following the twenty-eight-day program, seasonal jobs were opening up in a local tourist industry for the summer season. My adult child was offered a job that included a roof and three square meals a day. Perhaps a corner had been turned.

Shortly thereafter, my husband and I moved to another state. The furniture I had stashed for a sometime-place-to-live went to one of my clients at the mental health agency. I knew that no matter where I was, I could not secure sobriety for my adult child—that was out of my hands. But we had brought together something good, and I was tenderly optimistic. YES!

Well, no. When the tourist season ended, another downward spiral began for the one who I knew could be shown the way to health, prosperity, and a sky-blue life, given my good intentions. The tender post-rehab buoyancy evaporated. I was bereft, unnerved, and frantic.

NOW WHAT?

In the past I had been prescribed an antidepressant and anti-anxiety medication when I had grown frantic wondering how and if my loved one was surviving a particular crisis, but these circumstances were different. I was totally unglued after the perfect plan that I had waited years to implement, my *pièce de résistance,* had failed to save the day. There was no prescription for this. I needed human (and maybe more-than-human) intervention.

Years before, I had sought a professional hand up when my back was to the wall, but now I was on my own in a new community and didn't know where to turn. I needed help and needed it fast, so I dove into the Yellow Pages hoping to find a family support meeting. I had briefly attended a support group before we moved that was too loosely structured to be effective, but I felt it was a place to start. I tried a couple of phone numbers, and that evening I met with a group that I have grown to love and wholly trust.

The downward spiraling of my adult child would progress off and on for a couple more years. While I would never recommend living with addiction to anyone, I am grateful for what I was compelled to learn to survive my self-defeating and limiting behaviors, and to learn how to live differently.

I've given up my Princess Pleaser tiara. I am not cured of pleasing and don't necessarily want to be—getting along is good business in the world, and there is a vast difference between Princess-Pleasing and getting along. But now I know when "pleasing" is being driven by a hidden agenda, and I know when it is being delivered with a price. The price is always too high—not for the receiver, but for me. Call me a Princess Pleaser in Recovery. I'll never master it. This process is mine, and it is lifelong. I can live with that.

If I stay on my side of the street and mind my own business and pull my little red wagon, my adult child is free to do the same, and that is exactly what is happening. When I fall short or fall down, I know that I can get up. I know that I can help myself, and more often than not I do. If I can't, I have people and resources to call upon.

The world is less overwhelming, threatening, and unpredictable now. The sun can shine brighter and the stars are close. If I stop to smell the flowers and pet the dog and take notice of what is working in my life, I am less inclined to focus on someone else's stuff. I have plenty of my own, and that is just fine.

I can appreciate both of my children for who they are without continuing to raise them. They are freer, and I am free to spoil the amazing grandchildren they have given me.

Life is not perfect, but it certainly holds more possibility. The pressure is off when you are no longer driven to manage everybody and everything. That alone makes life a whole lot more promising.

I'm not responsible for anyone else's perfection, and I don't have to be perfect, either. Compared to where I have been, this is a state of grace.

• INTRODUCTION •

What Just Happened?

A misshapen moon cast a ghostly light in the house,

the same moon that had been round and whole

the night of your accident—your first DUI in 1993 . . .

—BV

WHAT JUST HAPPENED?!

It may have begun late one night when you were wrenched awake by a telephone call. It could have been any weekend, or the day before Easter, or on Thanksgiving. This awakening shows no respect for holidays or special occasions.

Your daughter or son made their one phone call from the county jail to tell you, Mom or Dad, that they had been picked up for driving under the influence (DUI). It might have been a patrolman, deputy sheriff, or sheriff who broke the news to you in what suddenly became your darkest hour as a parent.

As you stood in the dark with the phone to your ear, you pictured your young daughter/son, full of youth and vitality and promise, being held in a cell. Your mind raced with questions.

Is she alone? Is he safe? What kind of substance, or substances, was she taking? What happens next? Court? Fines? Counseling?

There is no parents' manual for this scenario. You have been blindsided.

Scarier would have been a call from the local hospital confirming that your daughter/son had been admitted to the emergency room. There was an accident and there were injuries. Your mind races beyond the initial questions.

How many people were involved? What was extent of their injuries? What legalities does this open up, and do I have enough insurance to deal with it? What are the next steps for my daughter/son?

The worst-case scenario is being summoned to the coroner's office to identify a body that could be the child you brought into the world or the child you adopted and have had dreams for since the day he or she came into your life.

Your girl. Your boy.

If you were contacted from jail or the hospital, you have everything to work with: where there is life, there is hope. Yes, your world has been turned upside down and shaken badly, but you will deal with it. Somehow.

Moreover, you are blessed, indeed, if your daughter/son's slide from substance abuse into the legal system proves to be a one-shot deal. After your child spends a night in jail, works to cover fines, attends DUI counseling or some kind of rehabilitation, is grounded for a good long time, or experiences some combination thereof, the ramifications of substance abuse kick in and he or she "gets" it. Everyone has received a nasty scare, but the bottom line is that the high hasn't been worth the hassle. You move through it together and everyone is wiser. Yay, you!

Some parents are not reprieved. One horrific altercation turns into another, and a pattern of behavior begins to emerge, with escalating personal risk and legal embellishments. Your daughter/son, meanwhile, is numbed, distracted, and bathed in illusions of well-being and empowerment as she/he turns into an addict. You, the parent, have no idea where she/he is, where you are, how you got there, or what to do in the alien world you have entered.

PARADOX NUMBER ONE

Attempting to usher a young person (or adult) entrapped in

substance abuse "over the hump" until he or she "gets it" will turn a well-intended mother or father into part of the problem, not part of the solution.

> **Our first instinct as parents has always been to protect our children. We guided them as toddlers away from the hot stove, the steep stairs, and the traffic in the street. Preventive guidance worked then, but no longer.**

Our first instinct as parents has always been to protect our children. We guided them as toddlers away from the hot stove, the steep stairs, and the traffic in the street. Preventive guidance worked then, but no longer.

Here's the cherry on top: while marshaling your best efforts against the chaos, you, Oh-Well-Meaning-One, are aiding and abetting a destructive course. Though every instinct you have exercised as a mother or father is driving you to do anything and everything to derail an emotional and physical train wreck, the "conductor" on this careening ride is the addict. The more you scramble for solutions, the more you, the parent, are enabling the addictive behavior to progress! Without realizing what is happening to you and your family, you have morphed into an anxious, frantic, crazy person, embroiled by a condition that you did not cause, cannot control, and cannot cure.

Welcome to codependency. You have now become part of the problem, not part of the solution. As if this weren't enough, your good intentions amount to sticking your nose into someone else's business—the business of the daughter/son you are trying to rescue. Even smoothing the rough spots for your child can provide only a temporary fix. Like applying a Band-Aid to a boil, treating the surface problem cannot reach what is going on underneath. The core of the problem continues to fester and grow.

PARADOX NUMBER TWO

You may be right about what you are thinking and feeling and saying, but you will be all wrong, because it won't change a thing.

You are hopping mad and have every right to be. You are sick, disheartened, and scared. You didn't bring children into the world to watch them wreck their physical and mental health, let alone break the law. *They should know better!*

Of course they "should," but that is one of the many platitudes that you will need to pitch. You can rant and rail about the predicament you have found yourselves in, but it will serve no purpose. Moreover, doors will slam. Darkness will fall between you and your offspring—and more than likely between you and your spouse as well. And silence.

A SINGULAR JOURNEY

The path that a parent walks with an addicted daughter/son is fraught with pitfalls that are unique to the parent-child bond. Your directive efforts can only assuage the madness for a short time. In the long run, you close off the avenues that you are trying desperately to clear. Your "being right" cannot guarantee anything except resistance. Your daughter/son is caught in a chemical quicksand that smothers and ensnares him or her physically and mentally, yet addicts will continue to do anything to protect what they have grown to need and want. Their addiction has evolved into a physical and emotional cocoon, isolating them from reality and responsibility. Mom and Dad have no chance against these odds.

Real change and healing can happen only when an addict (1) recognizes he or she has a problem, and (2) shoulders responsibility for his or her own healing. Parents must allow their offspring the power of choice by letting responsibility rest on their shoulders.

BUT . . . BUT . . . BUT . . .

How can I step aside and watch them destroy hope and possibility and alienate everyone who loves them?!! How can I NOT step forward??? Am I NOT to protect my own child?

Some people can't detach. One father could not help intervening in his heavily drinking son's life. He loved him deeply and believed in him, and wanted desperately for his son to succeed. If he wasn't covering bad checks for him at the local bank, he was putting money in his account so his checks wouldn't bounce. He knew the county judges and attorneys, and made sure he was in court for his son's appearances and sentencing.

He allowed his son to live at home and to use his vehicles, and hoped that by providing a "leg up" his son would be able to get a job and keep it and become independent and become the man his father knew he could be.

Father was there for every bump in the road. He adored his son and wanted the best for him. He thought he could eventually help him "over the hump" into a life of his own. He couldn't see that all the "help" he was doling out was actually preventing his son from coming to terms with his drinking and taking responsibility for his choices and his actions.

Year after year they went around and around together in a lethal dance, neither one knowing that he was sabotaging the other. It wasn't until the legal system intervened that the cycle was broken—for both of them. By then, the son was well into his thirties.

Which leaves the question, How and when does a parent step aside? That, Dear Heart, is why you reading these words.

FIELD MANUAL FOR AN ALIEN PLANET

This book is for you from one who lives in your world, written for all parents who love and dream for their daughters and sons who have become lost in addiction. These words are offered as a field manual to allow you to negotiate the treacherous landscape you have careened into headlong.

May you find guidance here for the steps you are being called on to take. May you find a measure of solace and a resource for your sleepless nights. May you learn from these words to develop muscles you never knew you had, to enable you (this is a good kind of enabling!) to widen your perspective beyond right and wrong, despair and hope, black and white. May you find guidance that grounds you where you are. And if you don't find what you need here, may you be led to resources that will help you on your journey.

FOR THE TERRITORY AHEAD . . .

Imagine yourself carrying a backpack filled with the good intentions, assumptions, platitudes, and clichés that no longer serve you where you are. You are going to dump them, and replace them with wisdom that works, from these pages. Much will be noted for you; I invite you to add your own. This guide is as expandable as you need it to be! Make it yours.

You are engaged on a battlefield. But the life you are fighting for is not for the daughter or son you have raised and are afraid of losing. The life you are fighting for is your own.

• PART ONE •

IT'S NOT ABOUT YOU

• 1 •

Planet Paradox

Where am I and how did I get here?

Surely there is something I could have known,

should have seen, done or not done,

for this not to have happened!

—BV

WHERE AM I, INDEED!

Suddenly nothing is the way it shoulda been, oughta been, coulda been.

Shoulda.

Oughta.

Coulda.

Throw them all out! None of these bums will serve you now, if they ever did. The watchwords for the world you have entered are ruthlessly simple: IT IS WHAT IT IS. Put this in the handy backpack you will empty of useless platitudes to be filled with functional "isms" for the road ahead.

"It" is the reality of interacting with your daughter/son in a way that will work as you tread gingerly together on a convoluted path. You will need a new set of benchmarks for this journey that are relevant to what you are up against. The only way to move forward through this landscape is to pay attention. What actually works may surprise you, especially if you persist in focusing on what *oughta* work. You must open yourself to allow what will work now for you and for your offspring.

I'D RATHER BE ANYWHERE BUT HERE!
You bet! But know this from the get-go: the only way off of Planet Paradox is through the landscape, with all its weeds and brambles, seemingly impenetrable woods, and fallen timbers.

Get comfortable being uncomfortable. No, you didn't bargain for picking up your daughter at the county jail, watching her face a judge in court, hearing fines and penalties and substance abuse treatment leveled, cringing as your girl is placed on probation—and seeing it all with your friends and neighbors the following week in the court record of the local newspaper—or, worse yet, on the front page. The scenario you find yourselves in was the last thing on your mind. Of course you would rather be anywhere else.

Get over it! Life in the world of It-Is-What-It-Is can be quite simple—deal with what is in front of you, one thing at a time. Support your daughter in court, meet with her substance abuse counselor, fill out paperwork for treatment and for financial assistance. You have plenty to do.

It's about what's happenin', Baby, not what you're afraid of out there in the woods or what might be coming down the road! Plant your feet in the here and now and take on the dragons in your path—*the known dragons.* Your hands are more than full without loading yourself up with maybes and unknowns.

WHERE IS THE NORTH STAR?

You're a lost ball in the weeds. You feel bewildered, betrayed, overwhelmed, scared, and shamed by what has befallen your family. This was never meant to happen on your watch. Mom and Dad were dotting all the I's and crossing all the T's. You were a mindful, vigilant parent.

What went wrong? Where do I go from here? How could I get there if I knew?

You have begun a journey that is, in fact, an open-ended process. You'll need a backpack on your way, but you will be traveling light. No frills on this path, Dear Heart.

THROW OUT RIGHT AND WRONG

Start by discarding everything that is nonfunctional, such as long-ago-and-far-away assumptions about "right" and "wrong."

You have to ask yourself, *Right and wrong according to whom?*

"Right" is what will serve you these days, not what "coulda," "shoulda," or "oughta" work.

YOUR BABY IS HISTORY

Your daughter "coulda" stayed home that night with Mom and Dad, or studied like she "shoulda," or rented a movie, or talked on the phone—you fill in the blank. Your son "shoulda" known better than to drink and drive, to keep company with scoundrels (and become one)—fill in the blank. She "oughta" be able to do better than this.

We didn't raise our children to end up in jail, court, or rehab. Your daughter had so much going for her . . . .

In twelve-step programs there are slogans that are the kind of thoughts you need. They can be life preservers to grab onto when you begin to sink under the weight of what your life has turned into as you have struggled to adapt to the addictive behavior of your loved one in a world you no longer recognize. Post them on the fridge, on the bathroom mirror, in the closet, on your steering wheel—wherever you could use a refreshing jolt during the day.

Mom, Dad, drop the platitudes. You need relevant words now.

SAVE YOUR BREATH

Driving home your "truth" at this time will fall on deaf ears, at best, and won't change a thing. You may be right in your thinking, but you will be wrong in the final analysis if your truth doesn't register with your daughter/son. And more than likely it won't. This is one of the most difficult "truths" you will have to reconcile with on Planet Paradox, my friend. Your child must come to "coulda," "shoulda," and "oughta" realizations on his or her own (and, maddeningly, in his or her own time!) for real and lasting change to be possible, let alone achievable. Your job is to take care of what is on your plate. Own your truths. Run with them. They are your property. Your offspring have their own, much different from yours.

THE FALLACY OF HINDSIGHT

Save yourself and your daughter/son a lot of grief by letting go of expectations and judgments from bygone days. Life seemed simple and predictable and on-track with All Good Things when your child was a scholar/athlete in school, and you were chairman of the PTA, a deacon in your church, president of your business and professional women's club, president of the Lions Club . . .

> **Save yourself and your daughter/son a lot of grief by letting go of expectations and judgments from bygone days.**

"What a lovely family," your community marveled. A perfect couple. Gorgeous children. And . . . and . . . and. . . . And here you are with your universe morphed into a nightmare.

Consider a farm couple with three children including two girls and one boy, who was the eldest. They had a nice little farm that was not big enough to support them all, but allowed her to be a full-time farm wife while he held a job in town that he worked at until he retired. He grew a sumptuous garden for the family, and she canned everything in sight, was a great cook, and kept a comfortable home. They were held in high regard in their church and in the community, the kind of neighbors you'd want down the road.

Their oldest boy did well in high school and played sports. He went on to college, he married a lovely girl, and they had a couple of little girls. The eldest daughter was a good student in high school, landed a good job after she graduated, and married her high school sweetheart, and they began raising two little boys. The youngest daughter was attractive and fun-loving, and did well in high school as well.

Somewhere along the way, the youngest daughter became derailed by alcohol, and it followed her into adulthood. Her engaging personality wasn't enough to hold a job or sustain a relationship long enough to call it one. Her parents wrung their hands and wondered what they had done wrong with their family, while the community whispered behind their backs: "Such a pretty farm," "Such good people."

Let it all go, folks! The Parents' Version of Hindsight is hardly 20/20. Life-as-It-Was probably wasn't as "on track" as it ever looks in retrospect, and certainly not the way it appears from Planet Paradox. More important, none of what you are going through with your child changes or wipes away your family history. Your strengths as a family and as individuals are not nothing. Draw on all of who and what you are. You'll need everything and more for the muscle and momentum to move forward and to keep from getting bogged down. Negativity is now your biggest foe, and it comes with plenty of cousins and hangers-on who will only sabotage you: depression, anxiety, and anger, for starters. *Pay attention!*

THROW OUT WHAT OTHERS THINK

Know this: you, Dear Heart, have not failed. Which goes hand-in-hand with forgetting about what other people think. This is a huge hurdle for you to move beyond! What can anyone know of what you and your daughter/son are going through, or what it is like to walk your path, let alone to face down the problems you are up against?

If the opinions of others ever mattered, which is open to debate, they certainly cannot serve you on Planet Paradox. People who are quick to judge—and there are plenty of them—will see only fragments of your reality. Genuine loved ones—to include friends and relatives—will not make assumptions about what they think they know, level accusations at you or your daughter/son, take sides, or make predictions.

The farm couple's youngest daughter would reach her thirties before she was able to come to terms with her addiction and enjoy a stable life, but it had nothing to with how much her parents worried over her or what the neighbors thought about them. It had everything to do with her deciding to make different choices.

WHO'S REALLY GOT YOUR BACK?

Keep company with those who have your best interests at heart, remain constant, and support you in whatever you are facing when you need it most. You will be amazed. The people who are the most steadfast may not be those who share your DNA. That's okay. Most people are petrified when they walk into their first twelve-step meeting. They are afraid they will have to talk, or be asked questions. This particular woman was no exception. She was a wreck when she came through the door, and had no idea what to expect.

The group welcomed her as a newcomer, and she listened quietly throughout the meeting. Before the closing, however, she shyly said her name and told the group, "I was scared to death when I came in the door, but I am so glad I did. You all get it. Nobody is judging me. You totally get it." Indeed. She has been coming back for two years.

Yes, you can back away from people who don't or can't "get it" and bring you down. Whether they can't help themselves or not is not your problem. The last thing you need is to be judged! Trying to persuade anyone to see things differently will only wear you out. Allow people their perspectives; you take care of your own.

Save your energy for the big battles. Align yourself with those who offer reinforcement. This may mean cultivating some different friendships, joining a support group, seeking out a pastor or church group. Whatever works for you now. And know that whatever benefits you will benefit your offspring as well.

ALLOW CHOICE

Cast off doubts, fears, predictions, and apprehensions about what may happen, is going to happen, or may not happen. You don't know where this is going. Moreover, *it is not in your hands!*

Get this, if you don't get anything else: the power of choice/change/healing lies in the hands and heart of your child. Period. All the strength and goodness you have poured into him or her since he or she was a baby is still there. *Own that.* Your power of choice is to allow your child responsibility for his or her own decisions on the path he or she is treading.

This is tough to "get." Your priorities as a parent must shift from what you can do to what your daughter/son must choose to do. This is a tough truth for a parent to accept. Use this for motivation: you are dealing with life and death—yours *and* your child's. In that order, Dear Heart.

SAY HELLO TO THE THREE C'S

Let go of guilt, blame, and regrets along with the "shouldas," "oughtas," and "couldas." All are mental noise. You must focus on IT IS WHAT IT IS. Put that in your backpack.

You are engaged in a process, a path, a journey that is open-ended. That's the hell of it. On the other hand, you are free to do the best job you can of taking care of what only you can manage—your own energy, your perspective, and unwavering love for your offspring.

And just HOW do I do that? I am the mother/father. If I raised this child, how can I NOT be responsible?

Unless you were actually procuring illegal substances for your daughter or son, or "using"—that is, partaking in—those substances yourself, you did not **Cause** their addiction. You certainly cannot **Control** their addiction, nor can you **Cure** it. You'll hear a lot about the "three C's" in twelve-step programs. They belong to our daughters and sons. Get this, Baby.

THE POWER OF ACCOUNTABILITY

Give your daughter/son latitude to choose his or her own consequences and his or her own victories. This is the only way that he, she, and you can grow through the process. As a parent it is torturous to watch your child angling toward a new pothole, a fresh legal entanglement, a shattered relationship, or all of the above. But you're not dealing with a toddler anymore. You, Mom or Dad, must equip yourself with the skill to back off. Otherwise, you are placing yourself in the middle of their situation.

Allow your daughter/son to be accountable.

MIND YOUR OWN BUSINESS

Yep. The only business you have is your own. You are tasked to morph your parental rescuing instincts into letting go of the management of your child and the consequences your child is facing. This is indeed a slippery slope to negotiate, and more than likely you will need an outside hand.

You may never know why your loved one landed on the self-destructive path of addiction, why they are putting their present and future at risk, why they are immersed in and causing others so much pain. But as a mother or father you are on the path with them. Get out of their way. Let them walk their walk, and you walk your own.

GET OUT OF YOUR OWN WAY

And what, you ask, does that have to do with anything? People, we have to get past our own egos.

Let's face it, most parents are probably guilty of thinking they can direct their children's lives better than their children can. Here is one of the grand paradoxes: that kind of thinking is right and wrong at the same time—right because we can see where drugs, including alcohol will take our children, and wrong because we think we can show them a better way if only they will listen to us.

In a life without addiction a parent might pull this off, but an addict will only listen long enough to get what he or she needs. Then your offspring's off again, on his or her way quite happily, leaving behind YOU, the bewildered and beleaguered parent.

Parents, if we get over our own fantasy of omnipotence, our children will be standing alone with their own choices. That is exactly where they need to be to "get" that they are running their lives, not Mom and Dad with all their big ideas (and resources). Which, in turn, puts parents where we need to be: making decisions for ourselves about what we need to be doing.

PLUPERFECT POSITIVE

Sometimes looking for the positive will be more than you can muster in the morning. You may feel paralyzed by what you are facing for the day, or what the day might bring. How safe to remain huddled under the covers.

Know that allowing for the positive isn't about turning into a Pollyanna, or grabbing for silver linings and happy endings. What impossible undertakings. This is about being real, about remaining open to what is and what can be revealed in the process of healing—for you and your offspring.

DON'T BE THE JUDGE!

Get off the bench! Don't be judge and jury for yourself OR for your daughter/son. Accept where each of you is at present—Planet Paradox—and shoulder the responsibilities that are yours to bear. Allow your offspring to shoulder theirs. Guard against hanging your hat on anything that is happening in your world. Stay loose. Allow for possibility, growth, and change. Otherwise you are inviting more booby traps onto your already cluttered path.

DON'T JUDGE YOURSELF

Here's a good one. If you're one of those people—and I am—who gets down on themselves when nothing is working, STOP. You may be doing the wrong things for the right reasons, but that doesn't make you a bad person. You just don't know enough to do the right things for the right reasons. Yet.

When we beat ourselves up we are stuck, stewing in our own juice. That's bad enough, and you don't have that kind of energy to waste! Lighten up on yourself, and you will be able to look at your situation with new eyes that can lead to better ways of doing things.

Be gentle. You need a little tenderness now. And Mom and Dad, you deserve it.

K.I.S.S. OFTEN

Enough already!

My college roommate from Ohio used a favorite Midwestern expression that I pass along for your backpack:

WHERE THERE IS LIFE, THERE IS HOPE. You bet. Run with that one. We may not know why things are happening the way they are, but sinking into despair is another way of becoming stuck. Possibility needs an open door, and if we're alive, Baby, we've got possibility.

Tuck this into your backpack, too: KEEP IT SIMPLE, SWEETHEART—K.I.S.S. Don't overthink. Don't overcomplicate.

The only way to eat an elephant is one bite at a time, so K.I.S.S. off whenever you can!

Travel light. Stay present. Be focused. Follow your North Star—It Is What It Is! Allow these words to ground every step that you take. If you do, I guarantee that you can move through the rough terrain.

The way out of the woods on Planet Paradox is to keep moving.

WHAT YOU'VE PUT IN YOUR BACKPACK:

• IT IS WHAT IT IS.

• WHERE THERE IS LIFE, THERE IS HOPE.

• K.I.S.S.—KEEP IT SIMPLE, SWEETHEART.

• 2 •

Your New Comrades

Never have I felt so alone.

I can't talk to anyone about what is happening to us.

How can they possibly know how to react

to a walking wound, without making it worse?

—BV

THIS WILL HAPPEN: You are at work, at the grocery, at church, or out walking your dog, and you run into a friend or neighbor. You're making chitchat, and, of course, the subject of children comes up and your friend launches into a litany of the wonderful things his or her children are doing these days.

"Oh, my John was just admitted to med school."

"Linda is going into the Air Force, and we are so glad after all the trouble she has had in the last few years!"

"Mike received a football scholarship to the University. . . .
Karla is getting married . . . . I'm going to be a grandmother!"

"What are your children up to these days?"

BE HONEST WITHOUT BEING EXPLICIT

OMIGAWD! A perfect nightmare, and you are totally NOT
prepared. Your mind races to come up with something that
won't be jaw-droppingly bizarre or reduce you to emotional
mush in the face of a seemingly innocent, everyday question.

What you don't feel like saying:

"Susan was stopped two weeks ago for driving under the
influence and has a court date next week."

"Troy got a break, and only has to do two hundred hours of
community service and six months on probation. We're hoping
he gets it this time."

"Eddie has been offered the choice of a year in drug court
or six months in jail at $60 a day. At least he can choose."

"We just finished completing reams of paperwork,
but the state is picking up the tab for Cynthia to go into
treatment."

You don't want to go into an incoherent meltdown, either.
So, how do you handle this?

First of all, understand that Planet Paradox is a parallel universe to the world most people operate in—that world you used to live in, remember? Few people can know, let alone respect, the path you are walking. So, you will want to tuck some innocuous responses for occasions such as this into that backpack you are carrying on your particular journey.

Know, for starters, that you are not obligated to be forthcoming about *anything* going on in your life just because someone asks.

What you might say:

"Oh, we're all getting along pretty well," then shift the subject. "Everyone stays so busy, we just try to keep up with them." Not bad. Certainly true.

"My daughter is having some challenges now, but we are working on them." Yep.

"How about them Dodgers?" Yay, team!

And you can always bring up religion or politics . . . .

Half-truths and generalities are no sin. You are entitled to wing it for self-preservation with a few handy words that you are comfortable uttering without feeling like a liar or an impostor. You also learn to give yourself an escape route to ease the conversation in another direction.

If this seems like a tall order, know that being a parent new to Planet Paradox is akin to being abandoned and isolated in an alien world. Some days it is all you can do to hold yourself upright, let alone engage in dialogue with another human. Other days, if you are asked anything at all about how you are doing, you may either clam up entirely or begin running at the mouth with far more information than an innocuous question warrants.

There is a middle ground between alarming extremes; you can be socially congenial without leaving yourself open to an emotional meltdown. To prepare yourself for being put in this position, it is essential to take care of YOU. Call it preventative medicine. More about this later.

I DON'T RECALL ASKING TO JOIN

Without aspiring or seeking to in any way, you have slipped into a hidden society that you never knew existed. You'd rather be dancing. Yep.

Gradually, you will run into other parents like yourself at school, through church, in your daughter/son's substance abuse or mental health treatment program, or through a self-help program for you such as Al-Anon, Nar-Anon, or CoDA.

Believe me, others are out there—just like you—like toddlers discovering other little people like themselves in the world. You will be filled with wonder that you are not alone. And you are not strange.

When you first meet other parents dealing with the same circumstances you are dealing with regarding your daughter/son, you will be cushioned by a community of like souls who understand exactly where you are and how you arrived there. Unofficially, you have been initiated into a club whose members hail from all walks of life, and who come in all sizes and shapes and from all educational backgrounds, economic circumstances, religious/spiritual affiliations, ethnicities, races, genders, and political persuasions.

There is no secret handshake with these comrades—though you know all about secrets and have been harboring plenty within your family. The bottom line is that no one is exempt from membership in this secret society. You and your fellow parents have had your worlds rocked to your foundations. The consequences of your daughters'/sons' addictions have caused seismic shifts in your families that are twisting all of your lives with heartbreak and mayhem.

THE GOOD NEWS

Oh, there is good news?

Yes! Among many humbling lessons that will float down around you on Planet Paradox is this: WE ARE MORE ALIKE THAN WE ARE DIFFERENT. Put that in your backpack.

Join the company and take counsel with those whose hearts have been fractured like your own. They are out there. Check your local newspapers and the yellow pages for support groups. Nar-Anon and Al-Anon are good places to start; the National Alliance on Mental Illness (NAMI) can help for those dealing with a dual diagnosis of addiction plus mental illness. Seek guidance from a rehab counselor.

It may not be much consolation at first, but you will soon learn that you have a lot more company on your journey than you can imagine. The world isn't made up of perfect parents with perfect children. We all come in shades of gray, and we live all over the map. Of the many gifts that will surprise you on Planet Paradox, this is a big one.

The burden you are carrying is a war wound; only a soldier who has fought on the same battleground can appreciate your experience. The challenge for parents in this war of wars is to trust that we have been placed where we are for a reason, and to seek support wherever we can find it. Wisdom will follow. It will.

Begin with your heart. If fear and anxiety for your loved one are overtaking you, seek the company of people who truly understand what you are going through. (There is much to be said for birds of a feather flocking together.) They will carry you along when you can't wing it yourself. They will help you see different ways of looking at and responding to your situation. As you begin to feel better about yourself, they will cheer you on, and soon you will become open to possibility and hope. Imagine that.

GO FOR IT!

Even if you find a good support group, you may need additional help. Recognizing this is not a sign of weakness; it is a sign of smarts.

Talk to a clergy member or a mental health and/or substance abuse professional—whoever and whatever resonates with you. Chances are they have seen it all and more, and you will be in good hands.

Consider medical intervention for yourself, as one woman did, when she couldn't sleep for wondering where her adult child was, whether he was sleeping out in the open somewhere, whether he had anything to eat, whether he was safe. She knew he had a duffle bag, and that was all. This happened during the Christmas season, which made the circumstances even more excruciating. How sad . . . how frightening . . . how unforeseen compared to Christmases past. How horrid.

She couldn't stop her thoughts. Her head was making her crazy night and day as she struggled with her home business. She felt she couldn't do anything right, and was behind in everything, everywhere she looked.

Everything and everyone was getting on her last nerve.

After weeks of going around and around and around in circles, it finally occurred to her to ask for help. She began with her general practitioner, who gave her a written evaluation to complete and then prescribed an antidepressant/antianxiety medication and a sleep aid. The doctor said it could take as long as six weeks for her body to begin to process it, but just talking to a professional about what was going on in her life gave her some peace of mind—that and knowing she had done something to help herself.

Getting more rest helped immediately. Gradually her head began to calm down and she was able to weather the uncertainty of what was happening with her son. Eventually she would know, but until she did she had to get through every day and every night.

So, Dear Heart, don't hesitate to talk with a health care professional about what is going on in your life. A thorough evaluation (oral and/or written) may be needed to prescribe an antidepressant or antianxiety medication that can help you through the rough spots and ease you into much-needed (and deserved!) sleep. You won't want to stay on medication forever, but judiciously used, it could provide physical relief for you to begin feeling better about yourself and move forward.

Most important, no matter how welcoming it feels to curl up in a safe haven and isolate yourself, DON'T! You are not alone in what you are going through. There is help to be found, help that you deserve if you need it. Reach for it, for YOU.

Just do it.

YOU NOW HAVE THESE IN YOUR BACKPACK:

• IT IS WHAT IT IS.

• WHERE THERE IS LIFE, THERE IS HOPE.

• K.I.S.S.—KEEP IT SIMPLE, SWEETHEART.

• WE ARE MORE ALIKE THAN WE ARE DIFFERENT.

• 3 •

Who'da Thought?!

A fellow twelve-step member, whose son was in jail,

said with a laugh, "The good news is that he has

three square meals a day and a roof over his head.

Makes you want to send out a Christmas letter!"

Our laughter was laced with reality;

jail is safer than the streets.

—BV

THE NEW "NORMAL"

In your new life, your son or daughter may:

- Lie unabashedly to you or to others

- Steal from you

- Steal from others

- Hock her/his belongings for cash

- Hock your belongings for cash

- Appear in court

- Be sentenced by a judge to

    — Serve jail time

    — Complete a rehab program

    — Pay restitution and/or court fines

    — Complete a year in drug court

    — All of the above

- Complete rehab, or fail to complete it

- Complete a year in drug court, or fail to complete it

- Continue to associate with drug addicts/alcoholics

- Serve extended time in jail

- Serve time in prison

- Relapse; relapse again

WHOA! Who would have thought that such events would ever become part of your daily life, and that you would need to take time off from work to deal with any one of them with the daughter or son you have raised?

This is beyond belief! How can this be happening to me, to my child, to our family?

But it is. So you take time from work to make a court date—you can't bear to see your child go through it alone. You fill out paperwork to have your daughter/son admitted to rehab. You meet with the substance abuse counselor. You take more time off from work (vacation or annual leave, of course) to attend "family week" for two and a half days . . . .

Welcome to your new "normal." While you have never felt more alone, you have more company than you think, with the epidemic of drug use among the young. Knowing and communicating with other parents on this same journey facing the same challenges will help you hold your head up and take steps that, by the grace of a Higher Power, will be forward. You are not the only mother or father tormented by very real consequences facing a daughter or son, consequences that were at one time unimaginable.

Know that you will become accustomed to dealing with the social and legal entanglements that have been thrust upon you. You will begin to roll with the punches that in your former life would have been incomprehensible. As you establish some measure of equanimity, you will develop a certain "black humor" with those who are going through it similarly. You learn to look on the "bright side" in a way that you never knew existed, let alone thought possible in your world.

"My son is in jail," your friend says, which may be followed by "At least I know where he is . . . and he's not using."

These can be strangely reassuring benchmarks, genuine pluses in your world. All is not lost. Where there is life, there is hope, indeed.

SURELY I'M RESPONSIBLE

Any reprieve you enjoy on the sunny side of Planet Paradox will be offset on the dark side with a nagging counterpart.

Guilt is a cumulonimbus cloud looming over the landscape.

I chose to have my child—and have raised him/her from infancy. Surely, in some way, I am responsible.

The twelve-step recovery support systems—which I highly recommend—will tell you that you didn't cause your daughter/son's disease, you can't control it, and you can't cure it. (You'll hear more about the three C's.) These folks don't truck with guilt, the first hurdle parents will encounter on Planet Paradox. The second megaleap is detachment (which warrants a chapter all by itself).

I would never assert that the path a parent walks is more difficult than that of a spouse or sibling or any other relative or friend of an addicted loved one. Any association with addiction by blood, love, or friendship presents staggering challenges. But the bond between parent and child makes guilt and detachment particularly confounding for parents, and is the reason you are holding this book in your hands. We are tethered forever to our children in ways that make detachment during a crisis feel like bald-faced abandonment.

HOW ON EARTH . . .

. . . can a parent wrap his or her head around what are blatant contradictions to the primal drives of parenting? *How do we NOT feel a sense of responsibility? How do we stop feeling it?* Above all, *HOW do we walk away from the actions of our daughters and sons that are life-threatening and/or criminal?*

Aren't parents meant to intervene, to act as caretakers in a crisis, to help our children through rough waters to a safe haven?

CAREGIVING AND CARETAKING

Quite simply, the mother/father heart has to be retrained. You get no free pass because you are Mom or Dad, as you would if your youngster were in the hospital because of accident or another illness.

There is a time and a place to be a "caregiver," which, as defined by one dictionary, means, "an adult who cares for an infant or child." Obviously, this definition works when discussing babies and young children, or the elderly and disabled. Care*taking* has a custodial implication, according to the same source, as in someone "temporarily performing the duties of an office."*

Caretaking that is open-ended is enabling and sets up a codependent cycle, as it did for the father and son described in an earlier chapter.

Our daughters and sons will never achieve healthy, autonomous lives of their own if we "take care of them" indefinitely—which too easily becomes the pattern with parents of an addicted daughter or son.

Our children must be handed the reins of adulthood while they are teenagers, and begin making choices with one hand, taking responsibility for the consequences of their choices with the other. Healthy adults exercise their power of choice in the best interests of themselves and society and have to assume accountability for their actions.

Addiction distorts the ability to make decisions and makes a laughing stock of responsibility. While a healthy young adult will embrace autonomy, addicts cannot. They have no

---

Dictionary.com Unabridged. Random House, Inc.
(http://dictionaryreference.com/browse/caregiver) Accessed May 31, 2012.
Caregiver, caretaker definitions used by permission.

autonomy because they are only grounded by a temporary fix, and the last thing that they can stand is to be held accountable. It's all about maintaining the status quo of their substance(s) of choice, staying even, and "keeping the edge off."

The only *modus operandi* an addict knows is to "keep on keepin' on" with whatever it takes to make his or her world work. Upsetting that apple cart is what rehab programs are designed to do. To begin assuming responsibility for his or her present and future, the addict cannot lean on *anyone* who will take care of him or her like "an infant or child," or perform, even temporarily, the "duties" another adult should perform for him- or herself. And that anyone means you, parents!

IT'S THEIR BABY, BABY

Get this: you, Mom and Dad, are not responsible for the choices of your addicted daughter or son. Period. Nor are you guilty by association for the mess he or she has made. Our children are responsible for the choices they make. The parents of addicts are challenged to let their children assume that responsibility.

The best thing you can do for your addicted daughter or son and for yourself is to begin educating yourself about how addiction works physically, emotionally, and genetically, so that you can begin making wise choices for yourself. Knowledge is power—your power. Interestingly, as you begin to empower yourself, your children will begin to take more responsibility for themselves. It's a fact. Someone has to do it.

DUH, everybody!

BLENDED FAMILIES

Parenting can be tough in blended households with his, her, and their children.

Whom do you support, how do you support, and when do you support? Or do you hold your tongue and back off?

All are valid and compelling questions.

Consider this wrenching situation: A couple in midlife was engaged to be married. Between them, three out of four of their children were addicts. She ran a family business in which her son helped when he wasn't into alcohol and prescription drugs. He lived at home. Her daughter, also an addict, was in recovery, living at home with her baby son. The groom's youngest daughter would be living with the couple after they married. His adult daughter was in recovery.

Talk about a "blended" family. When the son quit coming to work, stole from his mother, and wrecked her vehicle, the groom-to-be requested that he move out. The bride/mother wrung her hands; her son's biological father wouldn't take him in, and his friends had disappeared. There was nowhere for the errant son to go except rehab, which he refused to do.

All of these elements were in place, with a wedding approaching.

The first instinct of a spouse is to protect his or her partner. But what happens in a situation like this, when one's mate may have been reduced to a bundle of pain, anger, sadness, grief, anxiety, and raw nerves? Sleep deprivation has probably taken a toll, and he or she has withdrawn. That's probably on a good day. On an average day he or she has become irritable and snappish, ready to come out swinging at the least provocation and make it known in no uncertain terms that everything you say or do is getting on his or her last raw nerve.

It doesn't take long for partners to slip into a tit-for-tat relationship that brings out the worst in everyone. Before long, the only thing cooking between husband and wife is an anger that has taken on a life of its own, a dark being that is growing between the partners. And this is only the spouse factor. Imagine the effect on interactions with others in the household, with a daughter or son from a blended family, or children brought to the marriage.

No doubt you have heard people say that they didn't mind changing their own babies' diapers, but they had trouble diapering someone else's child. This pretty well sums up the dilemma of a blended-family parent, except the stakes are far higher than Huggies when it comes to living with a spouse's addicted child.

In this situation, the stepparent is in the untenable position of being outsider and insider at the same time, because the daughter/son in the throes of addiction is living in the home. Unless the stepparent elects to back off and wash his or her hands of the addicted one (which will put the marriage in jeopardy), the couple will need very good communication and a trove of trust between them if they are to manage the relationship. Both spouses absolutely must be on the same page, or the situation will implode, and everyone loses.

A family therapist is a valid option.

Our betrothed couple were married. The son went into rehab, was kicked out, and got into another program and left when he was offered work. Maybe he will stay clean this time.

What happens to the children in this blended family is unknown, but this couple will succeed together if they are open to each other about what each of them needs, and respect their common ground as well as their differences.

TALKING WITH CHILDREN

A grandmother struggled for the words to explain to her young granddaughter where her daddy was (in rehab), and why she hadn't seen him for three years (her mother wanted him to spend time in recovery).

Young children present the most wrenching challenge for parents or extended family who may be raising the child/ children of an addicted daughter, son, niece, or nephew.

Remember that a young child doesn't need too much clinical information or too many gory details—it's enough for them to know that Mommy has a sickness and needs treatment. They need reassurance that the reason their loved one is not around, or part of their lives, is not about them.

TELL CHILDREN THAT THEY ARE NOT AT FAULT. Tuck this critical element into your backpack. Don't imply that they are innocent victims; make it clear that they are not responsible in any way and that they are loved.

If the loved one is in rehab, you could say, "Mommy is not well and is getting help with her disease. She loves you, always."

Jail? "Mommy is not well and has made some bad choices. She is taking care of her obligations and straightening out her life. Know that she loves you, honey, she always loves you."

Alateen, which is for older children and teenagers, provides a safe place for children to talk about what is going on in their homes and share their fears and anxieties. They will also develop the language they need to process what their loved one is going through in terms they can live with. Many Al-Anon chapters sponsor Alateen groups, and they are listed in your community newspaper.

Don't let your anger or any lingering beliefs about addiction being anything other than a disease temper what you say when discussing

> **Don't let your anger or any lingering beliefs about addiction being anything other than a disease temper what you say when discussing a loved one's addiction with a young child.**

a loved one's addiction with a young child. Yes, you have a right to your feelings, and living with an addict tries the patience of the most saintly parent. But before jumping into discussions with children in these circumstances, know that nothing can be gained from running down an addicted parent or loved one to a child. Children will only feel more isolated and alone and different from their peers, whom they perceive to be living in happy, "normal" homes. And they will be utterly saddened. Don't go there with them.

If you are at a loss for what to say or how to say it, consider talking with the child *and* a substance abuse or mental health professional, or a spiritual advisor/counselor, if you have one. You will all be rewarded if you do so. The burden is removed from your shoulders to a professional trained in the nuances of communicating difficult truths under wrenching circumstances. Understand at the outset that you all may need to go more than once.

Watch and listen to your child or children. You may learn as much about how they are feeling from what they don't say as from what they do communicate. Remain present with them, and they will guide you toward what they need, when they need it.

Grandmother did all right. She chose her words carefully and paid close attention to her granddaughter as they talked. The girl was precocious, had spent a lot of time with her grandfather, who had died of complications of addiction, and already understood more about addiction than most people three times her age.

Grandmother and granddaughter communicated wordlessly at times, but when words were needed, as they were now, grandmother told the child that her daddy—who had gone to a treatment center—loved her, but that he was not well, and that he was getting help with his disease. The girl said she knew "the problem," as she called it.

"It has nothing to do with you," the grandmother said. "He always loves you."

No half-truths were told. No euphemisms. Grandmother and granddaughter understood each other and were closer for their talk. They hugged, and the little girl went out to play with her cousins. Enough had been said.

Honesty is the best policy with children—by the spoonful.

EXTENDED FAMILY

Your family may not include obvious addicts or recovering addicts among grandparents, aunts, uncles, and cousins, but it is more likely that your daughter/son did not arrive where he or she is in isolation. Addiction is a disease with a strong genetic component; in fact, science has now uncovered about a half-dozen genes that play a part in addiction. Read a few chapters in the recovery texts of any of the twelve-step programs, and you will be amazed. There is no one type of person who develops addiction. As a progressive disease, it can percolate for years—decades, even—without creating shattering drama. In advanced stages, however, it evolves with predictable and cataclysmic consequences.

Consider this family, in which four generations were impacted by addiction:

The grandfather drank alone most of the time. He drank not in bars but in his home, sometimes beginning the day with a shot of whiskey chased with a beer. He might have a beer with lunch and a shot of whiskey before his afternoon nap, and another round in the evening. Or more.

Family, and especially his wife, learned to stay out of the way of his dark moods and overbearing demands when he was in his cups, which was more and more frequently as he grew older. His wife began to rely on her sisters for support and a social outlet, and was very close to her daughters as well. The family agreed among themselves that the old man drank too much, but he'd always held a job, afforded a comfortable home, and had worked until he retired. When he wasn't drinking, he was warm and loving and told great stories, and was revered by his family.

His daughters could take or leave alcohol—wine, perhaps, but that was all. (One daughter didn't drink at all.) Beer and whiskey were the beverages of choice for his sons. Consumption ranged from occasional to habitual to heavy, though all held good jobs. One son would see his marriage come apart before all of his children left home. The family cut his wife slack when she left, because they agreed he had a "drinking problem."

Another son was married to a woman whose addiction became evident after their divorce. Their boys got into alcohol and recreational drugs in their teens, and veered into hard drugs and legal consequences as they grew into young adults.

Another son held a good job, ran a business, and raised a family. He consumed alcohol daily. When the marriage came apart, everyone was shocked. The question "How could this be?" resonated through the family and the community. *Their* son's youth was peppered by incidents with alcohol, and he was in his mid-thirties when the legal system mandated residential treatment.

Serious addiction began to show up in the next generation, the fourth, before graduation from high school.

Whether and how addiction raises its ugly head can depend on outside factors. A teenager may fall in with a drinking or using crowd and rapidly slide into full-blown addiction. Life crises—family upheavals including separation and divorce, death of a loved one, a parent's addiction, a broken romance—can throw a young adult into anxiety and depression, which, if prolonged, become inside factors that lead to "self-medication" with drugs and/or alcohol.

Regardless of when or how addiction occurs, parents are far more likely to encounter denial or an OMIGAWD response among family members than genuine sympathy or empathy— just what you don't need as you struggle to get real about what is going on with your child's substance abuse. Maybe they'll outgrow it, the family hopes. If we're honest about addiction, we know that they can't.

Few people want to examine in the light of day addictive behaviors that have been swept under the rug for a generation or two. These disclosures are scary and threatening. It is easy to have opinions about a crisis of the moment, but it takes real objectivity to see a pattern of behavior for what it is. Until addiction is acknowledged, it cannot be addressed as a disease. It is far easier to slather blame on the parents and their offspring as crisis after crisis accumulates.

Then there's the community—people who don't know the facts of what is going on with you but who have heard bits and pieces or read something in the local court news. The comments and innuendos are leveled at you from every direction until everywhere you turn you are seen as the "bad" parent of a "bad" child.

If you don't have the energy or resources to fend off the critics and tongue waggers in your family and community, tuck these words into your backpack when you're at a loss for how to respond to insinuations and accusations:

- THANK YOU FOR YOUR CONCERN.

- YOU ARE ENTITLED TO YOUR OPINION.

- WALK A MILE IN MY MOCCASINS AND WE'LL TALK.

And these four words:

YOU

HAVE

NO

IDEA

No kidding! Who can have any idea what it is like to live in the world you have entered—Planet Paradox—unless they have been there themselves?

Claim your dignity and you will find your feet. You will be able to help yourself, and this will begin to help your offspring.

DANCE TO YOUR OWN MUSIC

This is the most challenging footwork you will ever master. There is no right way to do it. Reach for a hand if you start to wobble: clergy, mental health professionals, marriage counselors, addiction specialists, and support groups. This is no time to hope you'll get better at it. Your child's life is at stake, and your marriage may be as well. Get the help you need as you need it and create your own protocols, solutions that will work for you and for your family.

Whether you want to or not, you are dancing all right. You may be making it up as you go along, but it's all right if it's keeping you together.

The poet Gary Snyder says it best:

Stay together.

Learn the flowers.

Go light.

YOU NOW HAVE THESE IN YOUR BACKPACK:

• IT IS WHAT IT IS.

• WHERE THERE IS LIFE, THERE IS HOPE.

• K.I.S.S.—KEEP IT SIMPLE, SWEETHEART.

• WE ARE MORE ALIKE THAN WE ARE DIFFERENT.

• TELL CHILDREN THEY ARE NOT AT FAULT.

• THANK YOU FOR YOUR CONCERN.

• YOU ARE ENTITLED TO YOUR OPINION.

• WALK A MILE IN MY MOCCASINS AND WE'LL TALK.

• YOU HAVE NO IDEA.

• 4 •

Don't Ask Me How I Am Today;
I Might Have to Tell You!

There are people I need to avoid when I'm having a rough day.

Their children are habitually stellar and they want to share the latest

details. If I get caught by one of them, I smile and listen politely,

and become pleasantly vague about our family.

Some days that's better than dark chocolate.

—BV

"Well, Hi! I haven't seen you forever! How are you?"

Did you have to ask? What do I say?

Time to take a deep breath. WHEW!

Remember the wisdom of grandmothers everywhere:
"If you can't say something nice, don't say anything at all"?

Be like a wise grandmother. Not everyone truly wants to
know how you are doing today, or any other day, for that matter.

More than likely you know the people with whom you can be frank and those with whom you can't, if you don't feel like spilling your beans. And that's fine.

You might just scare most people if you tell them that your daughter/son just received his or her third DUI and is spending six months in the county jail. Moreover, the thought of divulging the facts of how you may be feeling at the moment might be too scary for you to put into words or to hear out loud.

Don't "make nice" if you're not feeling nice. You can still be real. Find something innocuous to discuss if you can't muster being positive about your life at the moment.

"We've been working on the house . . . . Relatives we haven't seen for two years are coming . . . . I've been awfully busy at work and am doing a lot of overtime . . . . We've got the best garden this year . . . ."

Spare the drama. Serve up a little chitchat, and then turn the conversation around to the other person. "And what's going on with you all?"

If they seem puzzled by your response, it's okay. That is not your problem. You, Dear Heart, are in charge of what is "okay" for you and what is not.

Dodge the bullet. Some days you won't have enough stamina for chitchat or winging it socially. Stress has dulled your wits, and you're caught off guard. It's okay to be honest.

"You know, this isn't a really good day to ask. I'm dealing with a lot right now. How about you?" Puzzled reaction? Let it go. I've had to say this myself more than once, and it is liberating to be honest.

Some days you are sad. Some days you are mad. Some days you are in a daze. Some days you feel everything *but* okay. And some days you are strictly in over your head. It is all to be expected. On Planet Paradox you're in survival mode most of the time. What is totally "okay" is taking care of what you need to do, when you need to do it. Give in to it; ride with the tide.

Do what works! That might mean unloading on a genuine friend that your daughter/son was busted in rehab for possession of a controlled substance. Real friends will respect whatever you have to say or don't say. And they can be trusted with your pain, your uncertainty, and your anxiety.

Tuck this into your backpack to pull out for social situations that make you feel small, or less-than, as a parent: IT IS NOT ABOUT YOU.

The spiral your daughter/son has taken into addiction is about their choices. You are their loving mother or father, scrambling for how to be part of the solution, not part of the problem. Real friends will do their best to wrap their heads around it; most people can't. And so it is.

THE STUFF OF LIFE

One of the gifts of landing on Planet Paradox—and you will learn to identify many—is that you will become very grateful for and very good at living in the moment.

Savor every shred of goodness you encounter. Celebrate what is working for you each day. If you run into someone when you are not contemplating even the smallest ripple in your equanimity, you can say with honesty, "I am doing all right today, thank you. How about you?" You are not obliged to offer anything more.

Cultivate the fine art of paying attention to all that is going on around you—if you are surprised by an iridescent bluebird on your walk to the mailbox, if your cat climbs into your lap and curls up while you are watching the evening news, if the sunrise is especially colorful, if a soft rain is soothing, if someone does something kind for you for no reason. Relish the blessing. Focusing on the positive may sound corny, but it just may save your life. It will certainly save your moments.

Living with an addicted, loved child can consume all of our attention and energy. We can be swallowed by it, or we can reclaim who we are by focusing on the details of everyday living—grocery shopping, fixing meals, doing the laundry, paying bills, going to work, coming home to family at the end of the day. We are then more likely to make time for things we want to do for ourselves, such as going to yoga or walking the dog, and for things we want to do with others, like visiting an elderly relative, going out to dinner with our spouse, or watching our child's gymnastics meet.

Pay attention to the journey, not the destination. When your mind gravitates to the struggle and the heartache you are facing with your addicted offspring, remind yourself that the only constant is change. This, too, shall pass.

AN ATTITUDE OF GRATITUDE

One of the greatest lessons you may learn on Planet Paradox— which a group like Al-Anon or Nar-Anon will reinforce— is to be grateful for good things going on in your life. Begin keeping a notebook or journal to write down your blessings—

because that's what they are—when you meet them on your path. Read them on a good day. Read them on a bad day. Read them on a sad day. Write them down every day. A habit of writing down your gifts, the gratitude you have for your life, will serve you well in the short run and the long run.

During nights when you cannot sleep, don't lie in the dark twitching and turning. Get up and read your gratitude list; add to it. You will calm down and might even be able to get some sleep.

Gratitude strengthens the spirit and, like love, allows for more good things to flow into your life. You will reach a point when it does not matter which negatives are pummeling you. If someone asks, "How are you today?" you will be able to say, with all honesty, "I am well. Thank you for asking. And you?"

You will be able to do this. *Yes!*

If you pay attention, the path you are walking will change the fabric of who you are, make you more resilient, impact all your relationships for the better, and change your worldview. Corny? You bet! You can use a little "corn," Dear Heart. This is one habit you can afford.

Your daughter/son's addiction is about them; how you react to it is about YOU.

YOU NOW HAVE THESE IN YOUR BACKPACK:

• IT IS WHAT IT IS.

• WHERE THERE IS LIFE, THERE IS HOPE.

• K.I.S.S.—KEEP IT SIMPLE, SWEETHEART.

• WE ARE MORE ALIKE THAN WE ARE DIFFERENT.

• TELL CHILDREN THEY ARE NOT AT FAULT.

• THANK YOU FOR YOUR CONCERN.

• YOU ARE ENTITLED TO YOUR OPINION.

• WALK A MILE IN MY MOCCASINS AND WE'LL TALK.

• YOU HAVE NO IDEA.

• IT IS NOT ABOUT YOU.

• 5 •

The Abyss

Sometimes I am overcome with sadness.

The one I raised is disappearing into a stranger.

I don't know how to live with this loss

day after day, night after night. I am lost as well.

—BV

YOU HAVE PEERED OVER THE EDGE . . .

. . . and you have fallen, like Alice in Wonderland tumbling down the rabbit hole! You can't tell which way is up—but this is no rabbit hole and you are living no fairy tale. You plummet to the bottom and land hard. It is cold and dark. Your mantle is sadness and grief.

You've never been here before, and you've never been this low.

It's hard to even think about getting up again . . .

Where is up, anyway?

Is there an up?

Get used to not knowing where you have landed. It's all right. You may not know where "up" is for a while. You have fallen onto Planet Paradox through a hole in life as you've known it. Your challenge is to find your feet.

GOOD GRIEF

Grief colors your new landscape.

A first run-in with the law via substance abuse is nasty. You are sad; you are mad; you feel betrayed by your daughter/son. You hate to see him or her go through the consequences. But the wound can heal like a skinned knee from a bike wreck in grade school, with perhaps only a minor scar. If the "slip" morphs into addiction, however, your girl or boy of yesteryear disappears as innocence is shattered—yours and your child's.

Watching a daughter's or son's life unravel—the one you cared for as a infant, nurtured, encouraged, dreamed dreams for—is utterly sad. And as your sadness spirals downward, grief can become overwhelming.

It is all too unreal to get your head around. So much has been lost.

GOING IT ALONE

The "Solitary Man" of song and fable has nothing on you. You have never felt or been more abandoned. Or lost. There is nothing romantic about this brand of solitariness.

Since you feel as though no one can possibly know what you know or feel what you are going through, your instinct is to draw in and toughen up. You can muscle through this, yep. You can't get anywhere, though, curled up in a ball looking out at the world from the shadows.

You can tough it out, soldier on, but it won't serve you in the long run. Your best hope (perhaps your *only* hope) to dislodge yourself from the abyss is to become proactive. That is, move from a defensive position to an offensive one. You will need all the help and resources you can amass to navigate the terrain before you, which is why this book has been written.

WHAT DO I DO WITH ALL THE SADNESS?

Oh, my. How can you live with the utter sadness that has overtaken you and your family? How do you rise from the depths to which you have plummeted? You cry at the least little thing.

Some days you cannot bring enough strength to bear against the utter devastation around you. It may be all you can do to hold your head up, let alone to move about. That's okay. Just don't go numb, and don't settle into inertia.

Know that few of us can understand cognitively why we're walking the path we find ourselves upon, let alone the daughter/son who has dazed, crazed, and seemingly betrayed us. We are part of a grand design, whether we can perceive it or not. The work we can do lies within the parameters we are given. Some days this just has to be enough to go on. Trust the grand design. It is no lie.

My journey on this path has taught me that there are no accidents. How we respond to what happens to us, however, affects who we become. If you are sad, be sad. Cry your eyes out if you must. Some travelers I have met on this journey allot themselves a time frame to fully feel what has been pent up inside them—fifteen minutes, half an hour, whatever it takes.

Cry, thrash, yell—I've done that, too. When your emotions are spent, time is up. Inhale, take a cleansing breath, then exhale. You are done, Dear Heart. Time to move on.

DON'T JUST STAND THERE . . .

. . . or lie there. Inertia may overtake you at times, but don't get comfortable with it. There is always something you can *do.* Tuck this "truism" into your handy backpack. DO THE NEXT THING THAT LIES BEFORE YOU—as though bad news had not just walked through the door. Even if it is the most mundane task, you will be dislodging inertia. You continue to be a functioning, processing human being, and this is progress.

If you get a feeling of accomplishment by washing windows, do that! Work in the yard. Clean out the garage. Wax the car. Color your hair. Weed the garden. Trim your hedges. Tackle that chore or project you've been putting off because you never have time. Make time for something that has been waiting to be done. You will feel energized and noble, and you can use a dose of both.

Get out of the space you are in before you spiral downward into the mire. Stepping out of your comfort zone keeps you from getting stuck. Just do it!

STAY POSITIVE

Keep thinking positively, and know that you can avert your gaze any time—away from bad news, the latest drama, whatever is bringing you down. Start by homing into what is working in your life: physical health, a loving partner, employment, a comfortable place to live, or food on the table. Basics. Then refine your positives. Be specific and particular to you.

Do this exercise mentally when you find yourself in a downward spiral. Grab the good stuff around you. Or, once a day, make an appointment with yourself to write down those positives—in the early morning or before you go to bed. You'll soon realize this is no corny exercise. Rather, you will be sustained and empowered in a fundamental way.

There is always a situation or a story more complicated or sadder or more seemingly irresolvable than ours. An "attitude of gratitude" (as they say in Al-Anon) pulls us out of isolated thinking and links our humanity to another's. This is one of the treasures you will take away from Planet Paradox and carry with you forever. That is more than a promise. It is a fact.

BECOME YOUR OWN BEST FRIEND

Don't allow yourself to become vulnerable to every bump in the road. Be vigilant as you walk this new terrain by taking care of your heart, your thoughts, your energy, your love. Pay attention! Check in with your thoughts and feelings as you tread the edge of the abyss. Watch your step. The abyss will yawn, but it cannot pull you into darkness and loss and despair unless you allow it. How? By walking differently through the world as you know it now.

Inhale. Exhale. Quicken your step. Avert your gaze. Your lucky stars are shining in the night sky. Look for them. Look for the moon and sun. They are all shining. Love yourself, and you will be shining with them.

GET THIS!

Most parents don't have enough presence of mind to keep from falling into the abyss when their children have toppled over the edge, because we are wired that way. You leap after your tumbling one, right? Not on Planet Paradox! Here you pull back for your own salvation. It's your life that is at risk here. At some point, your child will have to manage his or her own fall.

Get your bearings. Hold the ground that is yours. The journey you are making may not look like anyone else's on this path, but remember that the terrain is yours. You may break new ground, and no doubt you will find yourself in a position to give another a hand along the way. But this journey is about you.

YOU NOW HAVE THESE IN YOUR BACKPACK:

• IT IS WHAT IT IS.

• WHERE THERE IS LIFE, THERE IS HOPE.

• K.I.S.S.—KEEP IT SIMPLE, SWEETHEART.

• WE ARE MORE ALIKE THAN WE ARE DIFFERENT.

• TELL CHILDREN THEY ARE NOT AT FAULT.

• THANK YOU FOR YOUR CONCERN.

• YOU ARE ENTITLED TO YOUR OPINION.

• WALK A MILE IN MY MOCCASINS AND WE'LL TALK.

• YOU HAVE NO IDEA.

• IT IS NOT ABOUT YOU.

• DO THE NEXT THING THAT LIES BEFORE YOU.

• 6 •

The Two-Headed Dragon

Addiction and mental illness present the most confounding challenge

I have faced. This two-headed monster will devour itself

and anything in its path. Yet it is in my path for a reason.

My task is to confront it, but how?

—BV

OH, MY!

Mental illness coupled with addiction delivers a double whammy. In mental health circles this may be called dual diagnosis, or co-occurring disorder. There are plenty of stigmas attached to each condition, loads of blame, and more than enough guilt for many lifetimes.

The following case is the most heartbreaking I have known of personally. The young daughter of a friend of mine was diagnosed as bipolar as a young adult. She was also profoundly alcoholic.

An attractive brunette, she was a gifted cosmetologist and artist, and the mother of an angelic little girl. When she was clean and taking her medications, she was personable and engaging, and obviously highly intelligent. As often happens, especially with young people, she would begin feeling good and "normal" and decide that she didn't need those meds, and go off them.

The drinking would start. She preferred hard liquor, especially vodka, but would consume anything she could get her hands on depending on how much money she had or could steal, which was often from her parents. Mouthwash or cough syrup from a discount store would do the job.

Her parents were at odds about what to do with her. Her father would stop speaking to her and forbid her to come to the house. Her mother would try to help her behind his back, give her money, pay her court fines, and look for yet another treatment program while her daughter was in and out of jail. Eventually, the young woman lost custody of her own little girl, who was sent to live with her grandparents—which was actually a bright spot in the scenario.

As cycles of using and abstinence continued, the young woman was in and out of the legal system. Eventually she became too tough a case even for drug court, and was ordered to complete a residential treatment program that lasted most of a year. It was very strict, and any infraction would send her straight back to jail. She was pregnant when she entered the program and gave birth to a little boy before she was released.

I was so hopeful for her when she came out. She transitioned into work as an aesthetician again, and for a while was living with her children. Within a year she relapsed again, and the grandparents had *two* little grandchildren to care for.

What talent this young woman had, and personality, and a good family behind her . . . .

CHICKEN OR EGG?

How can parents begin to assess what they're up against, let alone know how to approach a dual monster of addiction and mental illness?

The initial reaction for most parents is to ask ourselves what went wrong and when. Then we torture ourselves with what we *shoulda, coulda, oughta,* or *mighta* done differently. Isn't this is what we do best—figure out what went wrong and set about fixing it? We guide our children out of harm's way, pick them up when they fall, make the hurt place better. But this is no childhood boo-boo.

You may also torture yourself with a chicken/egg question of which came first, addiction or mental illness? This leads to the question of which do you treat first, and how do you treat it?

It all adds to your already-mounting anxiety.

You may search your memory for the fork in the road that you missed when your child took a turn you could never have foreseen.

Let go of the chicken-and-egg business and know this: addiction and mental illness must both be treated for total healing.

Treatment centers will support treating an addiction first. When the physical body is "clean," work can begin on the mental/ emotional dynamics that may be driving addictive behavior.

Where was I? Was I not paying attention? How could I possibly have missed it?

SELF-MEDICATION

Consider that one in twenty teenagers lives with depression of some severity, and that bipolar disorder, which presents with dramatic mood and energy swings, is often triggered in late adolescence by emotional trauma. Either of these disorders, added to the general fragility of adolescent emotions and hormone swings, offers a recipe for emotional crises.

Recreational substances have begun showing up in grade school and middle school. By high school, they can offer relief and solace for someone in emotional pain who wants it to stop, or to feel less bad, if briefly. It is good to feel good—yes, but it is a short hop from "feelin' good" into the swirling waters of self-medication and addiction.

YOU DIDN'T COUNT ON . . .

. . . this lousy piece of information: the emotional development of an addict is arrested at the time addiction begins. *Oh?* Yep, this means that a sturdy thirty-two-year-old can be conducting her affairs with the emotional maturity and judgment of a nineteen-year-old—accepting the kinds of jobs that she would have been glad to have in high school or college because they pay enough "to get by," living with parents, running with the same users she has known since they began using, and treating run-ins with the law as an annoyance to get out of, the inconvenience of the moment.

Addicts are invincible. They have all the time in the world. They don't see themselves as adults in their late twenties, early thirties, forties. Moreover, they have a breathtaking way of turning the concerns of their loved ones around: *And your problem is WHAT, Mom?*

Add this to your backpack: THEY MAY BE GROWN, BUT THEY'RE NOT GROWN UP.

AARGH!

Our gut reaction as parents is to rush to the rescue of our children, who will no doubt admonish us with "I'm an adult."

Really? Your gut says that your daughter/son is acting like a witless teenager. *So what's wrong with this picture?!*

The daughter or son you have raised has turned into an addict, and addiction has no power of reason. Nor does addiction arrive with a whit of respect or compassion for anything or anyone beyond the substance or behavior of choice. It maintains its hold with a voracious appetite, with no allowance for people, places, things, or special occasions.

Treat addiction as the brute that it is. Protect yourself from the behavior that has overtaken your daughter/son. The power behind it is beyond your control, reason, and emotional appeal. Period.

This brute has no conscience. It is apathetic. Treat it as such, but go on loving your daughter/son as you find out what it is that has a hold on him or her. Then you will know what kind of help is needed—medical, psychosocial, spiritual, or all of the above—and in what order.

KNOWLEDGE IS POWER!

Go to work on your own habits of self-sabotage: control, guilt, blame, and shame, which are rooted in a codependent dynamic that you didn't know you were feeding as it took on a life of its own.

Read! Read! Read!—about the cyclical condition of codependent behavior that arises between addicts and enablers.

Parents will benefit from reading about the many faces and manifestations of addictive behavior that can be found in twelve-step recovery literature. These titles are readily available from mainstream and recovery bookstores, as well as online.

Beginning with the personal histories of the founders of the programs, these books offer the outline of the program of recovery, followed by profile after profile of people in recovery from all walks of life, all income brackets, and all religious persuasions.

Learning about when and how drugs, including alcohol, have claimed people is eye-opening. The lives that have been wasted and all but destroyed, then reclaimed—not necessarily to preaddiction status but nonetheless saved—are tangible. When addicts begin to say no to alcohol or other drugs, their recovery begins and with it a new kind of living as long as they stay in recovery.

Knowing that addiction doesn't carry an inevitable sentence is important for parents. Our addicted children *can* heal from their habits, as others have before them. The stories, the pain, the setbacks, and the steps that have turned into miracles will stun and perhaps embolden newcomers on Planet Paradox. Real hope can emerge from heartache and ruin.

If your offspring suffers with mental illness and addiction, you are confronted with a confounding and complex situation. Parents need to understand the treatment for both disorders, and how professionals treat them separately and together. Understand what recovery will require for your daughter/son, and learn where to turn for help.

Co-occurring disorders are treatable when you understand what you're dealing with; then you go about addressing them both (though getting your loved one into treatment is another challenge).

At the outset, know this if you don't understand anything else: co-occurring disorders will not work themselves out or somehow "be all right." You must wade into the deep water with your daughter/son and find your feet to approach the confounding interaction of addiction and mental illness.

Consider seeing a family therapist, clinical social worker, or psychologist with your daughter/son. You may end up going together, but begin with yourself. You will learn that addiction is a family disease. Everyone has been impacted in some way and must take responsibility for his or her own well-being to heal self-sabotaging behaviors. You may learn that you have work to do that stretches back to your own childhood.

DON'T "DO" FEAR!

Take a brutal look at how you've arrived on Planet Paradox and you will be rewarded with new paths to consider, new directions to move in, and alternate ways to live.

Informing YOU is the first step to helping yourself and to approaching the two-headed, fire-breathing beast that holds your daughter/son in its clutches. There are plenty of resources available to clear your head of confusion, fear, and self-doubt. And you can find the facts you need, and the moral support you deserve, but you must take the bull by the horns and do the work.

Cowboy up. Start moving. Head out.

YOU NOW HAVE THESE IN YOUR BACKPACK:

- IT IS WHAT IT IS.

- WHERE THERE IS LIFE, THERE IS HOPE.

- K.I.S.S.—KEEP IT SIMPLE, SWEETHEART.

- WE ARE MORE ALIKE THAN WE ARE DIFFERENT.

- TELL CHILDREN THEY ARE NOT AT FAULT.

- THANK YOU FOR YOUR CONCERN.

- YOU ARE ENTITLED TO YOUR OPINION.

- WALK A MILE IN MY MOCCASINS AND WE'LL TALK.

- YOU HAVE NO IDEA.

- IT IS NOT ABOUT YOU.

- DO THE NEXT THING THAT LIES BEFORE YOU.

- THEY MAY BE GROWN, BUT THEY'RE NOT
  GROWN UP.

• PART TWO •

EXCEPT
WHEN
IT IS

• 7 •

The Shame Factor

When the specific legalities brought before the grand jury

were aired on the local radio station and in the county paper,

I could not help recoiling for the one I raised

from perfect babyhood—and for all of us who love this soul.

—BV

AFTER YOUR INITIAL SHOCK and horror have peaked, it is perfectly natural for this annoying thought to cross your mind:

What will people think?

PEOPLE!

Grandparents, siblings, extended family, neighbors, coworkers, anyone you are close to (or not close to) may read the local newspaper. They're all out there waiting to pass judgment on your daughter/son, and on your parenting skills or lack of them . . . or so you think. Your next dearest wish is—after wishing none of this had ever happened—*I hope nobody finds out.*

AND YOUR POINT IS . . .?

We all have "people" in our lives, but what you and your daughter/son are dealing with comes down to this: you have catapulted onto Planet Paradox and are orbiting so far outside of what anyone thinks of you, it is laughable.

Get this: your world is no longer their world; your normal is not their normal. Your good day is not their good day, and, in fact, might even be their worst day. And your bad day could be virtually unthinkable for them. YEE-HA!

Move on, Dear Heart.

BUT IT'S IN THE NEWSPAPER!

Here's the good news: Anyone who cares about you will have your best interests at heart and will not jump to conclusions about what they read and hear. They will not be rattled by the court news, nor will they pass judgment on you or your daughter/son. They will be concerned, and they will step forward when they can.

The friends you need and deserve will be there for you when you are ready to talk, when you need them beside you, and even if you don't need them. You have no explaining to do about anything to anyone. You are not obligated to discuss what you are not ready to share. True friends will be there for you, and you are truckin' with true, now. You deserve no less, but it took this kind of crisis to drive it home.

You would show up for your friends. They will show up for you.

Pull these words out of your backpack for the tongue waggers, the finger pointers, the naysayers, and the holier-than-thous:

YOU

HAVE

NO

IDEA.

Don't allow anyone to bring you to your knees! Step aside and keep on keepin' on. It's all relative—with your relatives and certainly with your friends, whom you will view with new clarity. And know that you will be making new friends on the journey you are taking.

KEEP IT SIMPLE, SWEETHEART—REMEMBER?

K.I.S.S. often! Here are some other suggestions for you to put in your backpack.

THROW OUT BLAME. You have nothing to be ashamed of, so don't even go there. You may be sad and sorrowful and grieving and angry, but don't blame YOU. Your daughter/son is the one who ingested drugs or alcohol. Your child put him- or herself on that path; you didn't. Dear Heart, you have more than a full-time job keeping your eyes on your own walkway.

THROW OUT BLAME. There's another item to keep handy in your backpack. Seriously, where does it begin and where can it possibly end? And what's the good of it, anyway? Water that has flowed under the bridge is gone. Get to know your mistakes, and stop repeating them. Let others be in charge of their own mistakes.

MIND YOUR OWN BUSINESS. Oh, my, you can't overdo this one. Tuck it in your backpack with THE ROAD TO HELL IS PAVED WITH GOOD INTENTIONS. Whip them both out as a reminder to back off when you find yourself stepping out of bounds. (And you will.) Doing the right thing for the wrong reasons can never be the right thing for long.

You will always have to backtrack and sort it all out. Stay on your side of the street, in your own backyard. You have plenty to occupy you there.

Time to get back to basics. The family you knew may have crumbled down around you, but you have a lot going for you. Lift your eyes and note all the blessings that are yours, basics unknown to millions of human beings across the globe: food, shelter, safety, people who love you, and people for you to love. Good health, if you are blessed with it; a job, if you are working; being able to pay your bills, if you can. Perhaps a pet that loves you unconditionally. A hot shower in the morning and a warm bed at night.

Start a list, and jot things down every day. Challenge yourself to see how long you can go without repeating anything. Food and family and shelter are gifts. Get humble about having the basics that are yours, and you will find a lot of luxuries as well.

Consider it a blessing to have family and friends who pay enough attention to be critical of you or your daughter/son—just don't buy into their criticisms. Thank them for their perspective and let it go.

Lighten up! We are all creatures of habit, and if you've been living with an addicted daughter or son for very long,

you have fallen prey to some powerful "stinkin' thinkin'."
Develop new thinking habits. If you can't come up with them
on your own—and you have no doubt felt so stuck that you
can't—get some help. Talk to your pastor, find a therapist, and
step up your visits to your support group of choice.

Delve into cognitive behavioral therapy (CBT). This
psychotherapeutic approach of talk therapy is directed toward
solving problems that are rooted in dysfunctional thoughts,
emotions, and behaviors.

The short definition of CBT is that it works by changing
our thinking—whether we tend toward negative thinking,
say, or black-and-white thinking patterns—which alters
our emotions and how we act. Even if external events do
not change—the addict in our lives continues using—if we
adjust our "stinkin' thinkin'" we will improve our response
to outside events, *which is all that stuff we can't control.* There
are all kinds of books and resources online, but a working
relationship with a cognitive-behavioral therapist could serve
you well.

Raise your gaze. Stop looking down. Look out, and look
up. Gradually, your perspective will change. Your focus will
shift. You will begin to notice shades of gray in your world

instead of black and white. Eventually your world will graduate to full color again.

Celebrate each small step. YES! Your gains are well deserved. You may take two steps ahead, three back, but on another day it may be three steps ahead, two back—or only one step ahead. Your gains are hard-won and real. Claim them. It will ease the switchbacks on a path that is never linear.

Go to a meeting. Hearing someone else's story can pull you out of your own drama. It may be a story like the one about a mother of five with three children in various stages of addiction (on various substances) and mental illness (bipolar disorder and clinical depression), with accompanying hospitalizations, rehabilitation programs, and legal issues including court dates, fines, sentences. She also ran her own daycare business—and, oh yes, was taking prerequisite classes to enter nursing school. Now there is a full plate.

Her former husband was a sometimes-recovering addict who was in denial about anything that had to do with her or their children, and criticized her at every turn. Somehow, this woman remained upright and breathing and maintained a wry sense of humor when she wasn't overtaken by everyone and everything imploding or exploding around her.

Some nights she would reel into the room on the verge of tears, sometimes she was in tears, and sometimes she was laughing at the latest convergence of preposterous events. Just seeing her there at all gave the group an attitude adjustment, and she always served up a rich blend of sympathy and wisdom, smarts and savvy. This was not a twelve-step program, but this group *worked* through unconditional acceptance and sharing and support, with guidance from a gifted clinical social worker.

There are many ways to take care of ourselves, and we don't have to do them all at once. Just keep your eyes open for what may help as you go along.

YOU'RE NOT THE CENTER OF THE UNIVERSE

Hmmm—sure feels like it when you are in the middle of a monstrous, life-threatening, full-blown crisis, with legal embellishments and fines, and . . . and . . . and . . . . Parents don't let their children become addicts . . . criminals . . . homeless . . . yada, yada, yada.

Tuck the three C's from twelve-step support groups into your backpack and keep them handy:

You didn't Cause *it.*

You can't Control *it.*

You can't Cure *it.*

Allow this triumvirate to penetrate your stinkin' thinkin'. You will find yourself removed as the source of everything and be able to look critics and naysayers in the eye. You will be able to say with equanimity, "This is a difficult time and we're doing the best we can," and you will be able to let it go.

You will no longer allow yourself to be blamed and shamed because you have stepped aside. It is not your game; it never was.

YOU NOW HAVE THESE IN YOUR BACKPACK:

• IT IS WHAT IT IS.

• WHERE THERE IS LIFE, THERE IS HOPE.

• K.I.S.S.—KEEP IT SIMPLE, SWEETHEART.

• WE ARE MORE ALIKE THAN WE ARE DIFFERENT.

• TELL CHILDREN THEY ARE NOT AT FAULT.

• THANK YOU FOR YOUR CONCERN.

• YOU ARE ENTITLED TO YOUR OPINION.

• WALK A MILE IN MY MOCCASINS AND WE'LL TALK.

• YOU HAVE NO IDEA.

• IT IS NOT ABOUT YOU.

• DO THE NEXT THING THAT LIES BEFORE YOU.

- THEY MAY BE GROWN, BUT THEY'RE NOT GROWN UP.
- THROW OUT SHAME AND BLAME.
- MIND YOUR OWN BUSINESS.
- THE ROAD TO HELL IS PAVED WITH GOOD INTENTIONS.
- YOU DIDN'T CAUSE IT. YOU CAN'T CONTROL IT. YOU CAN'T CURE IT.

• 8 •

Detachment

I simply cannot get my head around this! How do I "detach"
from my child who is going down in flames? I am not wired
that way, and I don't WANT to be wired that way. Addiction is
monstrous, but I don't want to turn into a monster, too.

—BV

You have GOT to be kidding!

How do you "detach" from a child you have raised?

How can I even think of it at a time like this?

How, indeed? This will be the most difficult challenge
you have ever faced with a daughter/son, and certainly the
most emotionally hazardous. You cannot kiss this boo-boo or
put a Superman band-aid over it.

You are tasked on Planet Paradox with reversing the
primal parental instinct to rescue your daughter/son in peril.

You must pull back when every inclination built into body and soul is to rush forward with protection and help. Instead, you must withdraw and accept that your offspring has been endangered by his or her own actions and allow him or her to shoulder the consequences. Ideally, you do all this with love.

Some love, you say. Some ideal.

For working purposes, let us call this pulling back from your child's circumstances "detachment." Essentially, you can approach it in two different ways. Neither offers a walk in the park or a rose garden.

TOTAL AMPUTATION

The simplest course is amputation—that is, you cut off all contact with your daughter/son. Good-bye and good luck. No interaction. No bailouts. No checking up, pleading, cajoling, or smoothing over, let alone covering up rough spots, anymore. You give them up to the life they choose, whatever that may be, by choosing to live your life without them.

A case in point: A mother had finally had it with her young adult son. She had raised him from her late teens as a single mother, so they had come through a lot together. He got into drugs in high school, and was in and out of the legal system.

Hard drugs were in the picture by the time he reached young adulthood, and she finally washed her hands of him. As far as she was concerned, she no longer had a son.

Some call this "black-belt Al-Anon," or "tough love on steroids," and it is not for the faint of heart. I call it breathtaking. Others just call it love.

Committing to the possibility that your daughter/son may or may not choose or sustain a path of recovery presents an unknown that few parents can accept. The only thing you will know for sure is that you have reached a crossroads where your paths must diverge. You can no longer make the journey with her or him. Your path together has grown too excruciating, maddening, and confounding for you to take one more step. You have already surrendered all the emotional and financial resources you have to give. You simply have nothing left.

Total amputation necessitates being at peace with walking away. To preserve body and soul, you withdraw from a life that included your daughter/son into a life of your own that may not.

I know people who have taken this route. Whether their parent-child interactions simply eroded to a place of zero contact, or they made an outright decision, or they became unequivocally and permanently pissed off, they opted for no further contact with their offspring—and, in one case, with more than one offspring, horror of horrors.

For one couple it became a matter of life and death between father and son. They would get into arguments that escalated into shouting matches, and the mother would be caught in the middle, placating them both. The biggest arguments occurred when their son relapsed and came home. The father couldn't contain his frustration and anger. Why couldn't a bright, sensitive young man see what he was doing to his life, and to them, his parents?

They kept trying to help. They would allow him to live with them on certain conditions: if he got help, if he worked to support himself and pay his fines, and if he stayed clean. When he got on his feet he would move out, and would do well for a time on his own, maybe for months. But there would be another relapse and he'd be calling his parents again or show up at their house with a fresh set of consequences that they would help him through one more time. He'd be with them for a while, then he'd move out, then he'd be back. The cycle went on for years.

Finally, there was a last confrontation. The father became so worked up during an argument that his wife was alarmed to see him turn a deathly white. Red in the face was one thing; this was different. Her husband had a heart condition, and she feared he would have a heart attack or a stroke. An alarm went off inside her and she heard these words: "It's time to go." This startled her, and she slept on it.

The next day she discussed her promptings with her husband. Finally, they agreed that the only resolution for them and their son was for them to leave. Obviously, he couldn't leave them for long. It just wasn't going to happen.

The next morning they packed a few things and drove across a couple of states to an area where they had enjoyed vacationing. They focused on finding a place to live and quickly did, then returned home, where they packed up everything they owned.

This mother and father, who adored their son, left without a word to him. It was the only way they could do it. They were gone. Period.

The couple always knew where their son was; he knew they had moved, but not where or how to get hold of them. Several years went by before they were in touch with him at all. Then they decided to call him. They told him that they loved him and believed in him, but disclosed nothing about their whereabouts and made no suggestion of getting together.

Afterward, they might talk with him a couple of times a year, but otherwise they left their son to his life and his choices as they created a life of their own, a good life with a recovery program. The son would hint at times that he'd like to visit, but they never allowed the conversation to linger there. They told him they loved him and believed in him, but they could not allow him into their world again.

Stress can kill; anxiety can kill; depression can kill. The stress and the unknowns of living with an addicted daughter or son can kill loving parents, well-intentioned parents. So, consider the wisdom given by every flight attendant to airline passengers before takeoff: secure your own oxygen mask first before helping another. Mom, Dad, that's YOU we're talking about.

Our couple saw their son just before he died in his early fifties. By that time he was no longer using illegal drugs, but his system had been too damaged, and he was abusing prescription drugs. The visit was sweet and sad. They knew their son would never be cured, that his health was fragile. As always, they told him they loved him and believed in him.

Two weeks later their son passed away. They had lost him to the disease of addiction, but he was at peace. They had seen him one last time. They would always miss him and always love him, but they were at peace for him. And they were at peace with themselves.

DETACHMENT WITH LOVE

The stark simplicity of "amputation" is not for everyone. If you simply cannot bring yourself to take that step, there are other ways to detach from your child's addiction that are less clear-cut and challenging, ways that are more diffuse.

You learn to live with the process in a world that is not black and white. You choose to walk with your daughter/son. You accept the potholes and switchbacks, blind turns, stonewalls, and the landscape clouded in a million shades of gray as you journey together.

Consider this particular process from the point of view of a woman who was raised with two generations of addicts, became an addict herself, and eventually fought her way into recovery. Her only child is not addicted to any substances, but her circumstances illustrate a particularly wrenching example of the complexities of detachment.

The woman's addicted grandparents had passed on, as had her abusive addict father; however, she still cared for her addicted mother, who had other severe health problems, in her home. She also cared for her addicted sister, who was paraplegic and lived next door. These are not the only family members she looked after who were addicts, but they were the most immediate with their needs, their demands, their anger, and their active drinking.

Living with the process of addiction and recovery is far more complex than cutting your losses, and no less hazardous, but this woman was doing it. She couldn't let go of everyone at once, so every day she compromised, winning here, losing there in a dicey dance.

Two recovery programs helped her manage her own recovery while living with a number of relatives who were actively using. Sometimes, caring for the emergency of the moment came down to this question that she would ask herself: *What can I live with?*

One night she wondered whether to check on her paraplegic sister, who had been drinking and might have passed out, to see if her catheter needed changing. The consequences could be serious if it wasn't changed. Should she intervene? Should she let it go? Her sister was drunk . . . that was *her* responsibility. What could she live with?

Which raised other difficult questions: How responsible should she be for the alcoholics in her family? How long is she responsible? When should she step in for someone in crisis who will turn around and use and abuse her?

She faces these questions 24/7, and she asks herself what she can live with at that moment. Sometimes she will step in to help; sometimes she lets them fend for themselves, like the night she let her sister ride it out alone. She remains the constant in their lives, balancing what she can live with and what she can't one day at a time.

The answers to these questions must be about you, Mom and Dad. What can you live with when it comes to stepping in for your daughter/son? What can you live with if you don't? What can you live with while you are trying to do what is best for you and for them, which may carry conflicting outcomes?

Some days you'll get an A+ when you let your offspring stand on her or his own. You hold your ground. You don't step in at all.

Some days you'll get a B+ and pay a cell phone bill so you can stay in touch, and your daughter/son can receive calls from prospective employers. Maybe you get a C- and pay a rent check. Maybe get a D- when you cave and bail your daughter/son out of jail and bring her or him home for a meal, a hot shower, and a night's sleep before considering the "What's next?" questions—you simply haven't the energy do anything else, and could use a night's sleep yourself, obtainable only because you know that your offspring is safe.

Do what you can, when you can do it, and don't beat yourself up over it.

If you can readily detach from your offspring's addiction, *Yay, you!* In my experience, however, that is not how newcomers arrive on Planet Paradox. They are more prone to panic and compromise and self-flagellation.

Plenty of literature exists on the Internet and in bookstores pertaining to detachment. Your most cogent resource may be veteran parents who have been sweating in the trenches for a while, particularly in twelve-step recovery programs for family members like you.

Point being: you can work detachment every which way and keep your balance, like the woman living with multiple addicted relatives, but don't be shy about reaching for help if you don't always earn an A+; you can't.

GET METAPHYSICAL

We can all learn something from the path we are walking,

whether or not we like the scenery. Self-mastery may be, in fact, why we are where we are, which is a constructive way of looking at it. If that kind of thinking smacks of hocus-pocus for you, however, draw on this oldie-but-goodie of your backpack: IT IS WHAT IT IS. Remember? Then pull up your Big Girl Panties or Big Guy Boxers and hike into the big picture.

Along your way you will be met by several bombastic yahoos decked out in flamboyant costumes with names like Unexpected, Illogical and Irrational, Confounding, Obnoxious, and Downright Perverse. Don't allow these bums to knock you off your path. You may feel alone in the challenges they are throwing at you, but you will be met by good company as well. Step over and join the good guys.

BUT . . . BUT . . . BUT . . .

It still feels as though I am abandoning my child. I don't think I can live with this.

I've never walked away before. How can I even think about pulling back at a time like this?

Detaching with love is not abandonment. It is steadfast vigilance for your own sake. The daughter/son you raised may be acting like a child, but childhood is done. Your job now, as a parent, is to let go of the responsibilities and consequences that are not yours. You have already given your all.

Your job, as an individual, is to take care of your precious self!

The addiction of your child is not yours to manage, only the compulsion you have to mend, fix, or ameliorate the situation. By learning to mind your own business, you begin taking responsibility for your broken heart, shattered dreams, and sleepless nights. Isn't that more than enough for you to handle?

The stress you have absorbed from your daughter/son's drama has morphed you into someone unrecognizable, a person who is impacting everyone around you—particularly your spouse and other children. No doubt your job and finances have suffered, and your self-esteem and self-confidence careened down the hopper along with your *joie de vivre*. You have learned to white-knuckle your way through the day, hanging onto whatever equanimity you can grasp. Even on your best day, this is no way to live.

Detachment runs a fine line. The mental, emotional, and spiritual agility you need requires self-care. Other people have accomplished this, and you can, too. One step, one moment at a time. Maybe someday you will be able to count days. Then years . . . .

CONSIDER AN INTERVENTION

If you are not ready to detach, if you still feel the need to *do something* by jumping into the mix, consider an intervention with your daughter/son.

There is a big "but" here: you would be wise not to go it alone with an addict. Get professional help before you initiate an intervention of any kind, and here's why.

We parents may know in our heart of hearts who our children are better than anyone, and built in to that heart of hearts is confidence that we also know better than anyone what is good for them. Well, that was all well and good way back when. As we all know, the picture has changed dramatically.

Intervention is an extremely intricate undertaking. Good intentions and great heart and decades of love may not be enough to intervene successfully in addictive behavior with a grown daughter or son. It is a touchy and potentially explosive process fraught with unknowns, because *you are not dealing with the daughter or son you raised!* You are dealing with someone deeply impaired, an addict/stranger who may bear a physical resemblance to your beloved child. Therefore, you are extremely vulnerable in this process, and so is your child. Moreover, with the best of intentions, you may be wholly misunderstood by the one you are trying to help.

When my family planned our first intervention, a "seasoned" parent in my support group smiled gently and noted, "This is your *first* intervention." I remember thinking to myself at the time, *You don't know how good we are; we'll get 'er done!*

Well, we got 'er done all right—the attempt to intervene—but we didn't *accomplish* a thing, even with a substance abuse professional present.

A second intervention was just nuclear family. We would cut to the chase. *Nyet.*

A third intervention was just Mom and Dad. We would handle it ourselves—but we didn't even come close.

To this day, I am appalled and dismayed that our loved one doesn't understand what we were trying to accomplish in any of the "interventions," let alone that we came together out of pure love to alter what we perceived to be a suicidal course. Our efforts were viewed as an attack. The net result was anger and alienation, and the conviction that we were bent on persecution and making life miserable for our loved one—the very things we were trying to avoid.

Interventions are viable, however, and they can work with the right resources at hand. From my experience, I would recommend that more than one kind of professional be present: a substance abuse counselor, family therapist, clergy member—whoever your daughter/son respects and who might garner their respect and hold their attention. Include other relatives besides nuclear family—aunt, uncle, grandparent, a trusted neighbor, a close friend—people who have resonated in a positive way with your offspring. Mix it up.

Unless your child can respect your intent in coming together, he or she will not be able to hear what you have to say. Only with this respect do you have a shot at being heard and an opportunity to initiate change.

Intervention is worth a thoroughly considered effort. And who better to attempt to break the cycle of addiction than a loving parent?

DON'T GO OFF HALF-COCKED

Many good books are available to help you structure an intervention. Go to the library and search the Internet. Don't be in a hurry. Do your homework and consult professionals in drug rehabilitation programs and mental health agencies if multiple diagnoses are present.

Intervention is worth a thoroughly considered effort. And who better to attempt to break the cycle of addiction than a loving parent?

DETACHMENT AS TRANSITION

Birth and death, the greatest passages of life, are transitions, and detachment is integral to both. Having given birth awake and aware, without anesthesia, I learned how mother and baby journey to the moment of birth together. From my experience with hospice, I know that the dying and the living must each reach the point of transition by letting go of each other. Both transitions involve physical and emotional detachment.

For our daughters and sons, addiction must "die" for them to move from dependence to autonomy—a true birth into a new life. For parents, the death of codependence frees us to focus on our lives by allowing our children to take responsibility for their own. By taking care of what we each need, parent and child sever codependent bonds and end the cycle of entrapment.

The transition from what we have known into a no-man's-land of unknowns can only be achieved by letting go. We experience grief and loss as habits die and we move from the known to the unknown, but we can do this. Moreover, we must do it.

As addiction and codependence are terminated, new life can emerge for parent and child, and between parent and child. This transition is the doorway to recovery. In a perfect world, everyone walks through that door together. More likely, parents and children travel on their own, but once the codependent bond is broken, a new relationship becomes possible. Moreover, it is probable.

"BEYOND DETACHMENT"

Not all addicts are pushed to the edge before they decide to get clean. And not all parents have to go to the edge with their daughters or sons. But when this happens, it is utterly terrifying.

A woman came into a support meeting blinking back tears. Her adult son was young and handsome and smart, and he was about to lose everything. He was drinking and he was using drugs. She also knew he was dealing drugs. She had refused to continue giving him money, and he was about to lose his apartment and his car. He had been missing a lot of work and was in danger of losing his job.

Losing the car seemed to be the last straw for the woman, his mother.

"I know it's just a material thing," she said, "but he loves that car. It is beautiful."

The car was the final break from the life he had and could still have. She was broken for him, and frantic over what it would mean, how bad it would get for him. She was standing on a cliff, looking over the edge, as life as he had known it fell away, piece by piece. How much would he lose, and would he fall over the edge himself?

Another parent on the edge was a father whose adult son was homeless, living with friends when he could or camping out. He "borrowed" the truck his father used for business and banged it up while transporting stolen property. He shot a bear out of season, and was only a few steps ahead of the police and the game warden. He had no income. His friends would feed him, and sometimes his father would feed him; sometimes he went hungry, but in that amazing way of addicts, he always managed to continue using.

"It's like he's asking to get locked up," the father said. His son had stolen from him in the past, but he wouldn't press charges against him.

"It's always about me with him, and I don't want it to be," he said. "I want the system to take him." He was afraid of what his son might do, but he was more afraid of what would happen to his son next.

This is a horrific precipice for a parent, and it is easy to become crazed with anxiety and grief. *How on earth do you pull back?*

You don't! Do you hear?

You stay put. You face your fear, your anxiety, and the terrifying unknown. You are Beyond Detachment here. What is called for is a suspension. You focus your thinking, your emotions, and your body on something beyond the precipice in front of you and your child.

You reach for your Higher Power as you hold onto this fact: no one can live on the fragile, frantic edge indefinitely. Something has to change; something has to give. That is the law of nature. You *will* be able to meet whatever changes or gives way because *something* has to change!

Now is when a twelve-step program can help you. Now is when a twelve-step meeting can help you. Now is when a twelve-step sponsor can help you.

Your child may, in fact, lose everything and go to jail, which is sad and frightening and an utter waste—but maybe not. That's the nature of change, Baby, and it just may become the point of no return for your daughter/son, the "bottom" that shows that the only way up or out is to change.

The disease of addiction is what it is. Whatever it takes to get through to an addict is whatever it takes. The precipice and the bottom may be exactly what he or she needs. The best thing that Mom and Dad can do is to let their child have it, own it, and begin to save his or her own life.

We may not be able to see the grand design around us, but when you arrive at the great falling away, that is the time to walk your spiritual path. You are not alone. Your Higher Power is with you, and with your child as well.

YOU NOW HAVE THESE IN YOUR BACKPACK:

• IT IS WHAT IT IS.

• WHERE THERE IS LIFE, THERE IS HOPE.

• K.I.S.S.—KEEP IT SIMPLE, SWEETHEART.

• WE ARE MORE ALIKE THAN WE ARE DIFFERENT.

• TELL CHILDREN THEY ARE NOT AT FAULT.

• THANK YOU FOR YOUR CONCERN.

• YOU ARE ENTITLED TO YOUR OPINION.

• WALK A MILE IN MY MOCCASINS AND WE'LL TALK.

• YOU HAVE NO IDEA.

- IT IS NOT ABOUT YOU.

- DO THE NEXT THING THAT LIES BEFORE YOU.

- THEY MAY BE GROWN, BUT THEY'RE NOT
  GROWN UP.

- THROW OUT SHAME AND BLAME.

- MIND YOUR OWN BUSINESS.

- THE ROAD TO HELL IS PAVED WITH GOOD
  INTENTIONS.

- YOU DIDN'T CAUSE IT. YOU CAN'T CONTROL IT.
  YOU CAN'T CURE IT.

● 9 ●

Codependence

I don't even understand the word.

I have only been doing what I have always done.

Suddenly, caring for my child makes me an "enabler," and

codependent, too—whatever THAT means. This is all nuts!

—BV

Is this a "woman thing"? 'Fraid not.

Codependence manifests in all genders, shapes, sizes, and ages, without regard for spiritual or religious preferences or economic circumstances. It is as psychologically sick as addiction and just as common—two illnesses walking with arms around each other.

You don't have to have an addicted loved one in your life to be codependent, but parents and spouses and loved ones of addicts often are. We can't stand to watch our offspring crash and burn.

Codependent behavior often precedes a partner or loved one falling into addiction. Take a personal inventory. Have you always been a fixer of problems? Can't stand a mess and simply must step in to clean up? Abhor seeing a loved one suffer, and rush to offer help or suggestions? Committed to being a pleaser, smoothing over, and making nice? Hate to hurt anyone's feelings? Hmmmmm.

Welcome to codependency. You have no doubt done one or more or all of the following:

- Lain awake wondering when (and if) your loved one would return home

- Furnished bail to get him or her out of jail

- Paid for the best lawyer you could find

- Covered his/her bounced checks

- Hid liquor (drugs), or poured it/them down the sink when you found the forbidden stash

- Made empty threats and not followed through

- Railed against addictive behavior

- Beaten yourself up for what you might have done to cause the problem, or what you should have done to prevent it

- Made excuses at school or at work for consequences of his/her behavior

• Lied for him/her

• Lied to yourself

Indeed, codependent behaviors stretch to the horizon. Some of us were wired to be pleasers and fixers from birth. Caring about any addict—spouse, offspring, relative, or friend—merely fine-tunes our natural bent. It also maims our best selves and who we were meant to be, and sabotages mental and physical health and any chance for happiness, let alone wholeness.

Codependent behavior literally distorts who we are, just as addiction can morph loved ones into people who are shockingly unrecognizable.

> **Codependent behavior literally distorts who we are, just as addiction can morph loved ones into people who are shockingly unrecognizable.**

COUPLES

You don't have to be a marriage and family therapist to know that mothers and fathers bond differently with their children. Although it is dangerous to generalize, the common wisdom that mothers seem hardwired to take a predominantly emotional and empathetic role with their children while fathers seem hardwired to take a more pragmatic approach seems to hold true. Parental roles may shift as children grow and parents become seasoned, but those initial bonds remain. This difference in biology can make detachment uniquely challenging for mothers and for fathers in distinct ways that are inherently instinctual. Unless you are alert to this dissimilarity, it can damage your partnership.

A mother's daughter/son who becomes addicted is a long way from the infant born into the world and held in arms, fed and cared for from day one. What the once-infant becomes as an addict is contrary to everything a mother knows of the person she nurtured with body, mind, and spirit. She didn't make junk. And just as it was with her little one whose fingers she held as she/he took first steps, a mother is psychically programmed to head off catastrophe, warn of an impending misstep, make better a nasty circumstance. Mothers seem to be made to help their children. We jump to fix "boo-boos" even after they have morphed into transgressions with adult consequences.

With a different biological nature, fathers may respond more pragmatically to their child's addictive behaviors. Certainly they are similarly vigilant for the welfare of wee ones, but addictive behaviors come with real-world consequences. A father may be inclined toward a more perfunctory reaction: *Stop it! Just stop! Get on with your life. Let us all get on with life.* This is an understandable reaction, but it has no more chance of success with an addicted offspring than does trying to "fix" the problem or soften the fall.

Healing from addiction does not proceed with clarity, nor does it follow a linear path. Urging an addict to "get over" herself or himself is not offering a solution—though that is exactly what we want to say, and where genuine healing can begin. The addicted "self" that must be "gotten over" *is* the problem.

Mothers may seemingly intuit their children's needs more from the inside out, whereas fathers may perceive who their children are more from the outside in. This difference in perspectives can create tensions, create fault lines, and insert "wedge issues" with potential for irreparable damage to a marriage. This is rough terrain, folks. A couple must be vigilant and honest about what is going on between them before they can stand together as parents and pull back from the urge to rescue or pacify their offspring.

You must take care of yourself, each other, and your partnership when journeying through Planet Paradox.

NOW WHAT?

Codependence has many layers, and can hail from decades before parenthood or addiction.

Some of us are wired for it from childhood experiences, and some by gender expectations.

Children may become casualties of codependence while growing up with addiction in a nuclear family or with multiple generations of addiction. As innate survivors, children learn instinctively how to stay out of the way of people who may hurt them. But the demands, the anger, and the mercurial behavior of addicted elders leave lifelong scars in young hearts. The double whammy is that the behaviors they perfected to survive as children will come back to bite them later in life, sabotaging who they are, who they can become, and how they conduct their relationships in adulthood.

Learn to identify the codependent behaviors in yourself and how they are impacting dynamics with your child. Typically, codependent people place a lower priority on their own needs by focusing on the needs of others. They may be driven by low self-esteem to "do" for everyone else but themselves. Parents who continue to take care of an addicted offspring may help on one hand, but on the other enable the addictive behavior to continue. A deadly cycle begins that takes on a life of its own.

Codependency is also about denial. A parent may be afraid to see what his or her offspring is really doing. There is fear—fear of what it means, fear of what will happen if a parent intervenes, fear of what will happen if he or she doesn't intervene.

There is bargaining when a daughter or son brings home consequences that a parent tries to "fix." A parent may try to control a child's behavior with threats: *if you do this, I won't do that,* or vice versa. You adjust a little here to mend a little over there, which enables the addict to get by one more time. That is codependence, which translates into enabling.

And there is narcissism—the self-gratification of a parent who becomes the rescuer on the great white horse, the solver, the one who placates, the parent who "understands" when the other one doesn't. Narcissism is believing unequivocally that we know what is best for someone else and we can make it happen if he or she will only let us. Mom, Dad, how well has that worked for you?

Parents are innately wired to direct and guide their children, but well-intentioned guidance turns narcissistic when it is driven by will. Oh, are we determined to save our addicted children from themselves. And oh, are we full of good intentions when we are desperate to save their lives. But desperation and good intentions and all the love in the world can't save an addict.

The underbelly of codependence is a passive/active manipulation: if I maneuver around the addict, I can arrange for the change that I know will help. This is empowering no one, because this kind of "rescuing" is about the rescuer.

See how convoluted codependent behavior is? It's like several animals entangled, with each trying to bite its own tail. Mind-boggling, yes, and it can take years to fully see codependence in our own behavior. Examine your own interactions with your child. Be objective about how you interact and when, and what your motives or (that nasty word) "agendas" are. I'd bet that what you see is eye-opening, if you are reading this book. Then get help.

Find a support group (several are noted in the back of this book). Talk to other parents walking on your path. Open up to any support system you have. You will not be turned away by anyone who has been where you are, and you need all the help you can gather to survive this journey.

HUMPTY DUMPTY

Life challenges always offer opportunities to learn, but no doubt you cherish a vision of what life was like before addiction shattered your family. Your children were just your children. Life was about work and school, little ones growing up, get-togethers with family and friends, and managing the vagaries of daily living. Life always had ups and downs, but it was, well, just life.

Now your life is barely recognizable. You have lived on the edge of fear, anxiety, desperation, and sadness. Then, by some triggering circumstance, you and your child and your family have fallen and have been shattered. You don't know how to get up or where to turn.

How do I do this? you ask yourself. *Can we put our lives back together? Is there a way back to life as it used to be?*

THE WALL

Some call it hitting bottom; I call it hitting The Wall. By whatever definition, you have reached a point of no return. There simply is no way back. And this, Dear Heart, is exactly where you need to be.

Hitting The Wall is the best thing that can happen to you and your daughter/son. There is no way around it or over it.

Fear will keep you rooted to the ground with your nose pressed against its rock face until you realize the only option you have: you must go through The Wall. *But how?*

With faith. With guts. And with strength and awkwardness. Like breaking the sound barrier, it is possible to emerge into a life on the other side of The Wall, beyond codependency, no longer emotionally tethered to the choices of another person.

Painful? Utterly. Breathe into the pain, as we are sometimes told to do in yoga. Look at fear, your quandary, the unknown, and follow your breath. The love for your daughter/son will go with you. You want all good things for your child. This is about your own momentum. You can no longer be bound by what your loved one may do or not do.

As you generate your own momentum you will reel on wobbly legs like the toddler you raised. You will wonder where you are going and what can possibly await you there. But you can muscle onward. You can get through this.

What matters now is that you are no longer lying in a shattered heap. You are not stuck. You will arrive where you need to be when you have stopped repeating the same behaviors that haven't worked while expecting a different result—a definition of insanity you hear at twelve-step meetings—and when you stop trying to force solutions to your child's addiction.

You have your own solutions; they have theirs. Period.

THE LAST GREAT PARADOX

Moving through The Wall is transition, a death, only you are dying into life—your own. It is also a birth—yours as well. And here is the best part: as you free yourself from the prison that is codependency, you will release your daughter/son to live life as their responsibility. Your daughter/son must reach The-Wall-of-their-making as well, and move through it in order to heal, but the timing and the choices are up to them.

Perhaps you will arrive together; perhaps not. But you can move into a new way of being where the immobilizing dynamic between you no longer rules who you are. You can live with joy and trust and honor and serenity. These are your birthright. And they will help you to pull together the fragments of yourself that have been shattered by grief and loss.

"All the king's horses and all the king's men" may not be able to restore you and your family to life as it once was, but, like a mended bone, you will have grown stronger in the broken places.

YOU NOW HAVE THESE IN YOUR BACKPACK:

• IT IS WHAT IT IS.

• WHERE THERE IS LIFE, THERE IS HOPE.

• K.I.S.S.—KEEP IT SIMPLE, SWEETHEART.

• WE ARE MORE ALIKE THAN WE ARE DIFFERENT.

• TELL CHILDREN THEY ARE NOT AT FAULT.

• THANK YOU FOR YOUR CONCERN.

• YOU ARE ENTITLED TO YOUR OPINION.

• WALK A MILE IN MY MOCCASINS AND WE'LL TALK.

• YOU HAVE NO IDEA.

• IT IS NOT ABOUT YOU.

• DO THE NEXT THING THAT LIES BEFORE YOU.

• THEY MAY BE GROWN, BUT THEY'RE NOT GROWN UP.

• THROW OUT SHAME AND BLAME.

• MIND YOUR OWN BUSINESS.

• THE ROAD TO HELL IS PAVED WITH GOOD INTENTIONS.

• YOU DIDN'T CAUSE IT. YOU CAN'T CONTROL IT. YOU CAN'T CURE IT.

• 10 •

Taking Care of Your Precious Self

"Being nice" has morphed into being real—

about what I want and what I don't want,

what feels good and what doesn't,

honoring what works

and letting go of what doesn't.

Life isn't what it used to be.

—BV

BACK TO GROUND ZERO

That's you, Baby. We cannot "parent" our daughters and sons through addiction. We need to develop a new paradigm of being ourselves that clears the way to be all that we are. Not Mom. Not Dad. Pure you.

Some benchmarks:

Love yourself enough to mind your own business. Period.

Fake it 'til you make it. Write these words on the inside of your wrist when you get up in the morning: Today I will act as if _____ (fill in the blank). Then do it.

Be the behavior you want to see in yourself. Be an actor if you must. Who cares? This is not being dishonest or malicious. You're not hurting anyone. You are developing mental muscles to overpower "stinkin' thinkin'," which is no small assignment. You're overriding old brain waves with new ones. Yes, you'll feel unnatural and off-kilter. Okay. You are getting rid of what no longer works and taking hold of what is functional.

GET OVER NICENESS

All our lives we have been schooled in the virtues of putting others first—by our parents, by our grandparents, by teachers and pastors and anyone else older than we were, which meant just about everyone. "Me first" wasn't "nice," and above all we wanted to be "nice" to win approval from our elders and to be accepted by our peers. "What about me?" was selfish and whiney, and we certainly didn't want to go there.

As we grew older, "nice" could secure careers, smooth marriages, win the attention of children, and make parents and in-laws proud. At least that's the way it seemed in the days of Goody Two-Shoes. "Nice" was a ticket to The Good Life.

Well, guess what? Life has changed. The Good Life is on hiatus, and Dorothy and Toto aren't in Kansas anymore. You are living in the alien realm of Planet Paradox where nothing looks or functions the way it ever did, and a good day is when somebody actually cares how you're *really* feeling.

"Nice" never served us well, but it took real upheaval to drive this home. There is nothing one bit nice about what you and your offspring are going through. Rehab, fines, jail— ARGH! "Nice" doesn't fit anywhere.

"Why me?" is beside the point. "What about me?" is laughable. The words you need are "What's working for me? What will be good for me right now?" Indeed. It IS all about you, Dear Heart.

GET THEE TO A SUPPORT GROUP!

One of your best tools will be talking with people who know what you're going through. They may not be people you've met before, but there are people whose eyebrows won't shoot up or their jaws drop at what is actually going on with you and your family. Your chances of running into these folks are better at meetings listed in the community news section of your local paper or online. Check them out. And consider that you may want to attend more than one group, like the mother of the young cosmetologist with a dual diagnosis who eventually became president of her local chapter of the National Alliance on Mental Illness (NAMI).

Twelve-step support groups form a worldwide fellowship for those affected by someone else's addiction. Call an AA or NA chapter if you don't see an Al-Anon or Nar-Anon listed in your phone book or online listings, and go from there. Someone will know where these family support meetings are being held or whom to contact.

Their programs are based on the Twelve Steps, and are about recovering from the twisted coping behaviors you have adopted while living with a loved one's addiction. Their premise is that we cannot change anyone else, but we can change ourselves.

The National Alliance on Mental Illness, (NAMI), has local chapters all over the country. Educate yourself about mental illness if your daughter or son is affected by these co-occurring disorders. Find out what kind of help you need and where you can find it.

There are groups for codependency for all manifestations of addiction—drugs (including alcohol), gambling, sex, food, shopping, and so on. Again, the phone book, your community newspaper, or the Internet will be the place to start. Do an online search for the organization and look for the chapter closest to you.

Support group veterans suggest attending six meetings before you draw any conclusions about whether the group will work for you. This is a good rule of thumb for any group. Follow your gut as you see and feel how a gathering resonates with you. Surprised to be "joining an organization"? You won't be the first, or the last, to feel this way. Think of it as trying before you buy.

Afraid to haul your "dirty laundry" out in front of people you don't know? Well, guess what—their dirty laundry looks more like yours than not.

READ! READ! READ!

Did I already mention that? I can't say it enough. Consult the Resources section in the back of this book for a range of books, for starters.

When I first attended my recovery support group, I took issue with their policy that we could only discuss group conference-approved literature in meetings. I was reading everything I could get my hands on, and this seemed restrictive.

There is so much literature out there that can help all of us, and we need all the help we can get.

I learned that that rule is in place for one reason only: to keep the meetings focused on the members and the stories that only they can tell. Discussions that wander off on tangents influenced by outside reading, treatment programs, and alternative philosophies divert the group from the work of focusing on their behavior and benefiting from the experience of others. Members lift one another by bearing witness to their respective journeys and by sharing what has worked and not worked for them.

As tempting as side trips into outside resources are, it is too easy for a meeting to spin out of control and take the focus off what the participants have come to share, and take away from the opportunity to benefit from hearing of another's experience. Seriously, there must be something right in a system that has been working around the world for decades. Members are free to share alternative resources with one another outside the meeting, or with a sponsor.

The Internet may be your quickest, most hands-on resource for reading material from different kinds of support groups. The library can also be invaluable. My advice is simple: leave no stone unturned. You never know what shred of material will open your mind, your heart, your soul to shed light into a dark place. Words can save lives—which is why I am writing here. Other writers have certainly helped save me, time and again.

NO ONE IS AN ISLAND

What appears to be a "group" is, in fact, a gathering of histories much like your own—of disillusionment, broken dreams, and hearts yearning to heal. You don't have to do anything at a meeting unless you are inclined. Look and listen. Ask what others are doing to help themselves, and what they are doing (and not doing!) for their daughters and sons. Check into the literature they recommend. Read everything you can.

The people you meet won't be strangers to you for long. Immediately, you will learn that you are not by yourself on this trail, you are not at fault, and you deserve better than you've been getting, which begins with taking care of yourself. Your insides will tell you if you've landed in the right place.

Cry if you must, share if you will, but most important, allow yourself to be held and beheld by people who "get it." You need safe haven now. In no time, you will relax and begin looking around with new eyes. And, by some kind of magical osmosis, the workings of the group will begin to work on you, from the inside out.

There is help and there is hope, but you need to cultivate a habit of reaching out. What you are reaching for are new tools for very different experiences than you ever expected.

TRUE FRIENDS

People who've known you pre- and post-Planet Paradox will fall into two groups: those who "get it" and those who don't, can't, or won't. You'll find out who is who real fast. Maybe friends who fall away will reattach as you heal your life, or you may lose them altogether. But the friends you make in a recovery group will be lifelong. You've helped one another through some of the roughest crises anyone, and certainly a parent, can face. The bond is unconditional.

Don't draw final conclusions about anyone (or anything) at this time. Just align yourself with whoever doesn't leave you feeling alienated or less-than. You need the support of your friends, not protection from them. True friends don't judge. They don't attack. They don't shy away or hold back. They are there for you, even when they don't "get it."

True friends know who you are and sense what you need. Those are the friends you need now, and deserve.

GROW A NEW VOCABULARY

You need a new way of talking with your daughter/son. And you need a new way of talking to yourself.

OH, I'M SO SORRY! WHAT ARE YOU GOING TO DO ABOUT IT?

Tuck these wise words from Granny Jean—a dear one I met in a support group for parents of children with co-occurring disorders—into your backpack. She would say this ever so sweetly when her adult son veered off into "woe is me" talk.

What are you going to do about it?

That is the question for all seasons, for each of us: *What are you going to do about it?*

Fresh words will lead to fresh thinking, which will lead to new ways of doing things. New action will change the tone in your relationship with your daughter/son and the energy between you. Your child will sense a difference in you even if he or she can't put a finger on it, and that will make a difference, slowly and surely.

Just as important as learning to talk differently with our daughters and sons is learning to listen differently. Don't keep your head cocked for what you want to hear. Sometimes the best thing you can do is to listen without anticipation. Their truth may be way out in front of you, something you have not heard from them before. Expect the unexpected.

GET OVER YOURSELF!

When we are wounded, our natural instinct is to draw inward and protect ourselves. But hunkering down for too long inside your own head invites inertia and depression. Shadows lengthen until the whole world is dark. Fear and anxiety begin chewing on your serenity like a pack of wolves. There is nothing like doing something for someone else to lift you out of your own problems.

Visit a nursing home whether you know anyone there or not. Offer to read to someone. Share some flowers from your garden. Gather the magazines you have finished reading and share them.

Volunteer for a hospice. Now there's an attitude adjustment. Consider what you would begin to do differently if you just learned that you have only six months to live.

Become a "big brother" or "big sister" to a child. Mentor a high school student. Roll up your sleeves at a recycling center if your community has one, or look into starting one. Join a community garden. Help in a food co-op. Pick up trash along the side of the road where you live. Put away books in the local library.

Wherever you are, there is always a shortage of hands; find something for your hands to do and it will help your head. You will rise "out of yourself," and guess what? Before you know it, you will be receiving much more than you are giving. Step out of your own shadows, and you will experience a seismic shift in perspective. Guaranteed.

BREAK NEW GROUND

Has there been a clown inside you all your life waiting to come out? Find a class or another clown to teach you how it's done. Enroll in a gourmet-cooking course. If you have a green thumb, earn a master gardener certification through your county extension service. Check out the continuing education courses in your area and sign up for something that has always interested you but that you have never investigated. Learn to play the piano— with a teacher or online. Learn to play chess, or perfect your game.

You may delight and surprise yourself with what you never thought you could do.

GET MOVING

There is no way to burn through angst like getting your endorphins pumping. Join a fitness club. Play racquetball (that'll do it!). Swim laps. Practice yoga, *chi kung*, or *tai chi*. Take lessons in ballroom dancing. Ride a bike. Jog. Walk. Return to sports you loved; join a softball league or volleyball team. Play basketball. Play tennis. Perfect your golf game—there's one that can keep you busy for a lifetime.

Physical activity beats back mental and physical inertia, which beats back the blahs, the blues, the mean reds, and the black blacks. Your head will be in a different place, and your body will thank you as well.

STOP MOVING

This is Planet Paradox, remember? Right is wrong and wrong is right and upside down is right side up.

You didn't arrive where you are overnight, and neither did your daughter/son. You won't travel through Planet Paradox overnight. Sometimes you just have to let the walk be what it is.

Remember the three C's of addiction—*You didn't* Cause *it. You can't* Cure *it. You can't* Control *it.* Slow down, and practice these three C's for yourself—take Caution, take Care, and add this one: CHERISH YOUR PRECIOUS SELF.

WHEN PARENTS ARE NOT ON THE SAME PAGE

It's tough going if you and your spouse do not see eye-to-eye on what is going on with your child, or simply cannot because:

- There is sheer lack of awareness.
- Nothing you can say is getting through no matter how you say it.
- There is outright denial followed by anger: *Not my daughter/son.*
- The parent in denial is also an addict.

Any of these responses presents a tough nut to crack if you are "getting" the picture and your partner isn't. You feel dismissed, thwarted, helpless, and at a loss for what to do with a daughter or son whose life is unraveling before your eyes. Withdrawing into uncertainty will only accelerate your feelings. And it is just a matter of time until real anger sets in and begins taking on a life of its own that grows between you and your spouse.

Such a separation of realities can erode the best of marriages, but this is not where your focus needs to begin. Begin with the problems overwhelming you. Take them apart one at a time and come to terms with what you need to do to address them.

Find a support group and go to a meeting alone if you have to, without fanfare. Don't plead or cajole or badger your partner. Just go. I guarantee that as soon as you walk through the door of a twelve-step meeting you will know that you are not crazy, making a mountain out of a molehill, or straining at a gnat. A cadre of people who know exactly what you are going through and why you are there will welcome you, and they will praise you for taking this step for yourself. This, Dear Heart, will be the beginning of your recovery.

> **Continue taking the steps you need to take, reading books, and seeking professional advice, and you will begin to change your reaction to the addiction drama.**

Continue taking the steps you need to take, reading books, and seeking professional advice, and you will begin to change your reaction to the addiction drama. As you change, your daughter/son will sense a shift in your perspective, and so will your spouse. As you become stronger, your daughter or son will sense a shift in the energy between you. They will have room to see that it is up to them now to paddle their own canoe out of the mess they have made of their life. Perhaps your partner will begin his or her own practice of personal caretaking, and you will begin working on recovery together; this is certainly a best-case scenario.

If you have to go it alone in your recovery, if you and your partner cannot see eye-to-eye on how to best handle your offspring in crisis, the two of you may have bigger problems to address than addiction. If your spouse is an addict, that is all the more reason for you to take care of what you need to, for yourself. Nobody else can or will.

Begin with you. Whether you are joined by those you love is not up to you; it is up to them.

YOU NOW HAVE THESE IN YOUR BACKPACK:

• IT IS WHAT IT IS.

• WHERE THERE IS LIFE, THERE IS HOPE.

• K.I.S.S.—KEEP IT SIMPLE, SWEETHEART.

• WE ARE MORE ALIKE THAN WE ARE DIFFERENT.

• TELL CHILDREN THEY ARE NOT AT FAULT.

- THANK YOU FOR YOUR CONCERN.

- YOU ARE ENTITLED TO YOUR OPINION.

- WALK A MILE IN MY MOCCASINS AND WE'LL TALK.

- YOU HAVE NO IDEA.

- IT IS NOT ABOUT YOU.

- DO THE NEXT THING THAT LIES BEFORE YOU.

- THEY MAY BE GROWN, BUT THEY'RE NOT GROWN UP.

- THROW OUT SHAME AND BLAME.

- MIND YOUR OWN BUSINESS.

- THE ROAD TO HELL IS PAVED WITH GOOD INTENTIONS.

- YOU DIDN'T CAUSE IT. YOU CAN'T CONTROL IT. YOU CAN'T CURE IT.

- OH, I'M SO SORRY! WHAT ARE YOU GOING TO DO ABOUT IT?

- CHERISH YOUR PRECIOUS SELF.

• 11 •

This Is Your Life

Besides detaching from codependence,

the biggest challenge I face is believing that all

is in divine order, that the Universe is working

as it should. I foresaw none of this,

yet I must trust what is evolving.

—BV

DID SOMEONE PROMISE YOU A ROSE GARDEN?

DANG! Shame on 'em, if they did. OOPS, if you bought into it.

Wasn't it just too easy, though, when our first little one was on the way and Gerber-visions danced before our eyes? As first-time parents, our hearts swelled with imaginings of what we would do for our babies, what we would impart to them—of who we are and where we've been in our lives, and where we might lead them in theirs. We cradled their tender bodies with dreams for them. And oh, the plans we made.

A few years of parenting later, it became obvious that we were receiving far more from our little ones than we were imparting to them. Then came the fun years of growing up—T-ball, gymnastics, school plays.

When we were catapulted onto Planet Paradox, our learning curve kicked into another stratosphere without our even realizing it. If you've been doing anything at all since you arrived, you've figured out that what we are learning because of our daughters and sons far exceeds anything we could have foreseen.

THERE IS A REASON FOR EVERYTHING . . .

Tuck this one into your backpack:

Regardless of your religious persuasion, life happens to us and we have to deal with it. So, there must be a reason for whatever comes our way, right? Sometimes we're responsible for it and sometimes we're not. But we still have to live with the whole ball of wax.

Working with life instead of fighting what we're given will beat back stress any time. "Woe is me" and "Why me?" never got anyone anywhere.

> **Working with life instead of fighting what we're given will beat back stress any time. "Woe is me" and "Why me?" never got anyone anywhere.**

The fact is, all experience arrives with something to be learned. Encased in the adamantine oyster shell of bitter experience is a pearl. Finding the pearl and figuring out what that pearl represents is the challenge facing parents whose children's lives have been ravaged by addiction. Our beloved daughters and sons are on their path for some reason, and we are on it with them. We all have something to learn; otherwise we wouldn't have landed here. Our mission on Planet Paradox is to understand.

Respecting where you are and where your child is sets a course—it's up to you to move into it. Get real. Get humble. Shoulder enough courage, and you will develop the grace to accept that you and your child are where you are meant to be. Acceptance leads to trust. Trust dislodges the inertia of sadness and despair, and there you are. Your momentum is faith as you trust that you are where you're meant to be for a reason.

. . . AND NO REASON.

That's for the backpack, too.

We can also accept that what has happened to our families doesn't have to be comprehensible. Your family is in chaos, but remember the three C's: You didn't Cause it. You can't Control it. You can't Cure it. This triumvirate opens a door to equanimity where healing can begin.

Parents are challenged to shut down an erroneous belief system that says "good" parents should be able to control and direct their children. Our work is no longer on the outside; it's an inside job that begins with the mind-set that good parents can control their children and uphold what is right and just and true for them. Our daughters and sons are challenged to sort out what is driving them from the inside to reach for their particular form(s) of addiction, to shut down that response, and to make another choice.

As we all begin to give up control of what lies outside our purview, we free ourselves to live with integrity and awareness in our own backyard.

Develop the art of living in the here and now, and you will begin to trust your life again. "Shit doesn't happen," folks. Life happens for reasons that we may not see, but that are ours to accept and master. When no reason appears, the habit of trust will grow into, guess what? Faith.

BE A MOVER AND A SHAKER

Your family has landed in the psychic boonies. Become a steward of this environment you are inhabiting, for however long. Know where your feet fall. Feel the ground pushing back. Breathe the air around you. Read the sky. Know when gale winds and golf-ball-sized hail threaten to flatten you and everything you hold dear. Be prepared by getting smart.

The environment on Planet Paradox has one positive characteristic, at least, and it is this: when you pay attention to the things that will take care of you where you are, your surroundings will begin to change. Confusion will diminish, clouds will disperse, and light will filter down and begin to warm your bones. Your world will change as you begin to change, and so will your relationship with your daughter/son.

After attending a support group for a year and a half, a mother related that her son, who had just relapsed, remarked, "You seem really good, Mom. You're different." Indeed.

Shake off habit and make room for fresh air. You can heal yourself, your life, your love, your spirit, and your home when you let go of what doesn't work anymore, what doesn't serve you. And when you do, this is a given: the life that opens around you will make any "rose garden" promised by someone else pale by comparison—because the roses come from you.

THE ART OF THE SILVER LINING

Looking for the silver lining to any thundercloud doesn't require Pollyanna eyewear. Silver linings are about vision, not sight. Vision is about perspective—through, around, over, and under—and paying attention. In searching your own thunderclouds, remember this, and put it in your backpack: THE ONLY CONSTANT IS CHANGE.

No matter how dark the canopy hanging above you, it is the nature of clouds to move. They shift up and down and sideways. Pure light will always filter through, because it always exists above if not below. This is the reality of clouds and thunderheads. And it is the reality of Planet Paradox.

Become a silver-lining chaser. RAISE YOUR GAZE. Look up instead of down. Step out of the darkness of what-used-to-be, no matter how comfortable it seemed. Your world has exploded beyond anything that has ever existed for you before. With every step away from what was once your comfort zone, you move into possibility. It's another world out there now, and it can be your best ever: the world of NOW, not THEN.

Light will find you through those thunderheads. That, Dear Heart, is the nature of clouds—and of change.

IN PRAISE OF THE LEGAL SYSTEM

You've got a silver lining here, too. Hard to believe, isn't it, since no parent ever envisions their daughter or son behind bars for one night, let alone days . . . or months . . . or years. But sooner or later, that's the route that addiction often takes. Pull up your Big Girl Panties or Big Boy Boxers and adapt to it, Mom and Dad.

WHAT?

Indulge me here, and you'll make it through a fundamental truth: society has a legal system in place for a reason that is grounded in humanity. Courts and detention centers and prisons are not in place solely to corral career criminals and enforce restitution. They enforce consequences that can lead to changed behavior and new lives.

Many a parent has been able to reach a wayward daughter/son by taking a hard line, but tough love can roll off another addict like water off a tin roof. If your daughter or son is forced to serve time of any kind, accept it. This is the last thing you wanted for him or her and for you, but focus your attention, instead, on the individual you raised. All the love and guidance you poured into your child as he or she was growing up still live beneath layers of addictive habits.

LEGAL CONSEQUENCES

A court sentence from an objective judge can jerk a hard line on a young adult, enough to get his or her attention in a way that a parent cannot. This kind of real-world feedback, as tough as it may be, may register with your offspring and lead to real change. The focus becomes how he or she is going to get through it. Not Mom or Dad, who aren't around to help.

And here's another aspect of "getting real" to consider: there are worse things than being in jail. Dear Heart, living on the street can be far more precarious and dangerous. So are driving drunk and selling drugs and prostituting to survive. Don't kid yourself; those things can and do happen.

The long arm of the law can put an addict into court-ordered rehab, enforce community service, or flat scare the hell out of a "good kid" whose habits have spun out of control.

The sooner your daughter/son realizes that their behavior will continue to lead them into court, the better. So, take heart, parents. Possibility is built into the legal system for those who need it, and that just may be the right thing at the right time for your daughter/son. Getting help and getting straight, with legal clout behind it, can be a good deal in retrospect. And it just may save your child's life.

Pull this "ism" out of your backpack to tuck under your arm if you find yourself looking through a plexiglass wall at your offspring wearing an orange jumpsuit as you talk to each other by telephone: WHERE THERE IS LIFE, THERE IS HOPE.

If your child has been handed a sentence, he or she has also been handed an opportunity. Jail or prison is tough going all the way around, and redemption may seem a long shot. But genuine change happens in detention centers and jails and prisons every day. Your daughter or son has the stuff within to push through habit and addiction and to reclaim who they are, because you gave it to them.

Let your child do his or her time if necessary. Visit. Call. Give support and love. Believe that the system can work, and turn it over to that Higher Power greater than you are.

What your friends and family and anyone else on the outside looking in think is totally beside the point. Your child is alive, and he or she has been given an opportunity to change. YES!

YOU NOW HAVE THESE IN YOUR BACKPACK:

• IT IS WHAT IT IS.

• WHERE THERE IS LIFE, THERE IS HOPE.

• K.I.S.S.—KEEP IT SIMPLE, SWEETHEART.

• WE ARE MORE ALIKE THAN WE ARE DIFFERENT.

• TELL CHILDREN THEY ARE NOT AT FAULT.

• THANK YOU FOR YOUR CONCERN.

• YOU ARE ENTITLED TO YOUR OPINION.

• WALK A MILE IN MY MOCCASINS AND WE'LL TALK.

• YOU HAVE NO IDEA.

• IT IS NOT ABOUT YOU.

• DO THE NEXT THING THAT LIES BEFORE YOU.

• THEY MAY BE GROWN, BUT THEY'RE NOT GROWN UP.

• THROW OUT SHAME AND BLAME.

• MIND YOUR OWN BUSINESS.

• THE ROAD TO HELL IS PAVED WITH GOOD INTENTIONS.

• YOU DIDN'T CAUSE IT. YOU CAN'T CONTROL IT.
  YOU CAN'T CURE IT.

• OH, I'M SO SORRY! WHAT ARE YOU GOING TO DO
  ABOUT IT?

• CHERISH YOUR PRECIOUS SELF.

• THERE'S A REASON FOR EVERYTHING—
  AND NO REASON.

• THE ONLY CONSTANT IS CHANGE.

• RAISE YOUR GAZE.

• 12 •

Am I Okay Now?

Sometimes I all but look over my shoulder

when I'm having a good day,

wondering if it's okay to feel good.

Then the least little thing will send me

hurtling to the ground. I am fragile, precarious, and it is unnerving.

—BV

THE "NO" PART FIRST

Life as you've known it is over. Your family cannot resume its preaddiction configuration once the addict is no longer "actively using," as they say in recovery circles. It just doesn't work that way. You have been changed forever, and so have your daughter or son and your entire family. Your OKAY has turned into living with the WHAT IS of recovery for you, and for your offspring.

Recovery is each day, for the rest of your days.

LET'S TALK ABOUT RELAPSE

Must we?

Get real. There are no guarantees that any of us can respond flawlessly all of the time—not you, Mom and Dad, or your daughter/son in recovery. That doesn't mean you sit around waiting for the other shoe to drop, or that you need to fly out of bed if the phone rings in the middle of the night (there's a knee-jerk habit to break). It means that we're all human. Life will happen, and you can't respond flawlessly all of the time.

Sometimes it is you, Mom and Dad, who will relapse or disappoint yourself and your daughter/son (or your spouse). Just because we know what we need to know and what we need to do and not do doesn't guarantee that we'll come up with the right response at the right time.

Don't let it rock your world if you catch yourself wondering, *Why did I fly off the handle at him? Why did I pay that fine? Why didn't I let her go to court by herself this time?*

We may disappoint ourselves with enabling behaviors, and most of the time we will know when we are doing it by the sick feeling in our stomachs. Don't put yourself down with self-recrimination. Open your eyes and look at what is happening for what it is: a controllable reaction (ours) to an out-of-control condition (addiction). Easier said than done? You bet, or you and I wouldn't be here.

Your daughter/son may relapse or disappoint as well. Sometimes they may appall you; sometimes they may scare you. Their steps are not linear any more than yours are, and no one can always be on point. (Otherwise, in my humble opinion, none of us would even be here—we'd be raindrops or snowflakes or butterflies or some other form of natural perfection.)

No matter how maddening or frightening recovery seems, we can accept that we can all get to where we need to go in order to heal, and give ourselves up to that journey. As we learn to trust our own momentum, we will trust momentum for our daughters and sons.

The course of recovery will never run straight and smooth into a sky-blue life on the horizon, just as *coulda, shoulda,* and *oughta* are no longer fence posts along our way. Your life is not about achieving perfection and a movie ending; it is about the journey.

Recovery is a river. Swim through it, roll with it. Don't grab for a rock in the rapids; lie back and feel yourself being supported by the current. Focus on the clouds overhead if the scenery rushes at you hard and fast. "Roll along, mighty river, roll on," as the folk song says.

Allow the river to take you where it needs to go. You are where you need to be, and you are all right. The river will carry you. Tune in to your Higher Power, however you perceive it to be. Float, knowing that your child has his or her own Higher Power as well.

Accept recovery as a dynamic process. You are all growing, acquiring skills to face what must be faced, to accept the unacceptable, and to move through brokenness. Affirm that process every day.

Trust the journey. And be realistic about it.

KNEE JERKS AND HOT BUTTONS

Knee-jerk justice is so-o-o-o-o seductive! Feeling white-hot rightness in the moment is exhilarating, all right, but a feeling doesn't guarantee rightness or appropriateness. Self-righteousness is pure "stinkin' thinkin'" and goes nowhere good. But here's the real issue: addicts have built-in sonar detection and will shut down all communication with the slightest ping of "holier than thou." Whether you can tell or not, they are already beating themselves up more than you ever could. Don't add to it.

Knee-jerking always fouls the best intentions. You may feel right and you may, in fact, *be* right, but if your best intentions are not heard by the person you want/need to have hear them, the sum of your effort is a big zero.

Put YOU CAN BE RIGHT, AND STILL BE WRONG in your backpack, if it's not already there.

Hot buttons and triggers become tools for someone else's agenda. We all have them, but addicts have a genius for finding and working them to get what they want. Parents are easy targets for their children because we are programmed to help. We are oh-so-eager to step up to the plate, fix everything, smooth everything out. We long to "make nice" so that sky-blue life can happen for our children and our families, for the hypothetical rose garden to bloom. So we don't always pick up on what our clever offspring are doing when they are actually working us over. Any addict is a master manipulator, even—and especially—our precious children.

Our work on Planet Paradox is to tune in to the dynamics of what goes on around us, then to choose how it will affect what we say, think, and do. Don't be seduced by being "right." Conserve your energy for your own affairs. A white-hot self-righteous reaction is a lie. Look below the surface of instant truths for the wisdom in the moment. You will find it waiting for you in your gut. Be responsible for your own responses, and the truth you speak will be right for the right reasons. Only then do you have the best chance of being heard.

NOW THE "YES" PART

You are better, and you're getting better every minute of every day that you stay focused on your behavior and not on someone else's. Bingo. When you develop the knack of using practices that actually work, you will feel better, if only in increments.

It's good to feel good, and we're empowered when we feel better. That, friends, is what our addicted children have been taking substances and pursuing behaviors for: *feelin' good, feelin' great, feelin' empowered.* That's some elixir, the Great-I-Am, the I-Can-Be, and the I-Can-Do-Anything. Only you're not taking a shortcut. You are inching toward your own "feelin' good" with the mental and emotional and spiritual mojo of who you are. This is what all humans want. When you reach that sweet spot on your own, nothing and no one can take it away from you.

GOOD-BYE, CHICKEN LITTLE

You are not abandoning your child-in-need if you've hauled yourself out of the dumps and stopped wringing your hands. You don't need to feel guilty for living your own life instead of your daughter/son's. Whether or not the other shoe drops is not up to you. The sky doesn't have to fall. This is one cloud cover that you can hold up on your own.

> **Stand on the solid ground you've earned, and treasure it.**

Stand on the solid ground you've earned, and treasure it. Celebrate the baby steps you begin to take—they are, in fact, huge. Walk your walk, mind your business; look up instead of down. And do spoil yourself a little along the way. As the hair-color folks like to say, "You deserve it."

YOU ARE WHERE YOU ARE

While paradox may have cropped up in your perspective throughout your life, now your very feet are set upon it.

They always will be. You have hit The Wall and made your way through into a world that has changed forever, and you have survived. You have grown into a different person, a different parent.

This upside-down world of twists and turns and switchbacks of Planet Paradox will always be part of who you are, and you've earned your ground, your territory. You can walk, jog, and run on it, lie upon it when you are weary, and arise from it renewed. You will be swept by wind and rain, blanketed with snow, warmed by the sun, and illuminated by the moon and stars. Your footwork is just fine now. You can negotiate anything and remain centered.

You are beyond OKAY. You are mighty and fine.

RECOVERY AS SPIRITUAL PRACTICE

By now you may have already seen the light. Religion per se has little or nothing to do with your healing process, or your child's. The condition of spirit has everything to do with it. Belief in God is not required, but a belief in a Higher Power of your understanding will be the turning point in how you get along. Why? Because WE'RE NOT IN CHARGE. That's for your backpack. Something beyond our comprehension is in place.

Getting in touch with whatever that is for you will bring you to your feet.

Whatever the particular thing is that lifts you out of the sadness, loss, loneliness, and grief you feel for where you and your loved one are isn't important, but it will make all the difference in your world if you access *something* that allows you to release those feelings. Maybe it's calling a friend who is working on his or her own recovery. Maybe it's spending time in nature. Maybe it's swimming laps until you notice that your head is beginning to clear. Maybe it's taking your mind off of everything with a movie, music, painting, writing, or dance. Maybe it's a hot bath by candlelight, or meditation, yoga, or *tai chi*, or getting a massage. Maybe it's attending church or talking with your pastor. Maybe it's taking time to experience the grandeur of the moon and stars or the rising or setting sun.

We're not the center of the universe, but we are the center of our world. So do whatever shifts your perspective and lightens the load on your journey. Spirit is the "wind beneath our wings," lifting body and mind and emotion. Spirit will help us heal. Spirit gives us flight.

Many have said that we are spiritual beings having a human experience. Invest in Spirit and you tap into all that is and all that you can become. There you will find the heart and soul of your recovery.

And, in these words, IT'S NOT ABOUT ME, EXCEPT WHEN IT IS ABOUT ME. Amen to that, Dear Heart.

Now go take care of your Precious Self.

YOU NOW HAVE THESE IN YOUR BACKPACK:

• IT IS WHAT IT IS.

• WHERE THERE IS LIFE, THERE IS HOPE.

• K.I.S.S.—KEEP IT SIMPLE, SWEETHEART.

• WE ARE MORE ALIKE THAN WE ARE DIFFERENT.

• TELL CHILDREN THEY ARE NOT AT FAULT.

• THANK YOU FOR YOUR CONCERN.

• YOU ARE ENTITLED TO YOUR OPINION.

• WALK A MILE IN MY MOCCASINS AND WE'LL TALK.

• YOU HAVE NO IDEA.

• IT IS NOT ABOUT YOU.

• DO THE NEXT THING THAT LIES BEFORE YOU.

• THEY MAY BE GROWN, BUT THEY'RE NOT
  GROWN UP.

• THROW OUT SHAME AND BLAME.

• MIND YOUR OWN BUSINESS.

• THE ROAD TO HELL IS PAVED WITH GOOD INTENTIONS.

• YOU DIDN'T CAUSE IT. YOU CAN'T CONTROL IT.
  YOU CAN'T CURE IT.

- OH, I'M SO SORRY! WHAT ARE YOU GOING TO DO ABOUT IT?
- CHERISH YOUR PRECIOUS SELF.
- THERE'S A REASON FOR EVERYTHING— AND NO REASON.
- THE ONLY CONSTANT IS CHANGE.
- RAISE YOUR GAZE.
- YOU CAN BE RIGHT, AND STILL BE WRONG.
- WE'RE NOT IN CHARGE.
- IT'S NOT ABOUT ME, EXCEPT WHEN IT IS ABOUT ME.
- MY HIGHER POWER LOVES ME EVERY DAY AND EVERY NIGHT, BEYOND ALL DAYS AND NIGHTS.

• EPILOGUE •
Little Victories

There are moments when every precious detail of what is good

and whole and real stands out in high relief.

I tack those moments to my mental bulletin board for when I need

them. I've found them before; I can find them again.

—BV

OUR LUCKY STARS . . . .

As these words were being written, the offspring of a well-known and very wealthy Hollywood family was receiving a sentence for possession and conspiring to traffic in drugs (to be sold to our sons and our daughters).

Correction: HALF of the mandatory sentence for conspiring to traffic in drugs (to be sold to our daughters and sons).

Members of the family plus friends and Hollywood icons wrote the judge some two dozen letters attesting to the young man's character and prospects for rehabilitation. Terms such as "caring," "considerate," and "worthy human being" were attached to the wonderful person their loved one could be, and who was "now taking responsibility" for actions that can span an adult life. Prospects for rehabilitation were viable because of family support, with no one letting anyone down "this time."

All are valid statements to render in love and hope for our daughters and sons.

One mother wrote to a judge outlining her son's history of substance abuse—not to obtain leniency, but to provide a full picture of his history of alcohol abuse before his sentencing for a DUI. The state in which the most recent DUI had occurred had a nasty legal loophole that allows a DUI more than three years old not to be counted for current sentencing. Therefore, a fourth DUI could be counted as a third, or a second. She was convinced that her son needed treatment after accumulating several DUIs. All it would take for him to receive a minimal sentence would be a savvy defense attorney to represent him in order for him to get off relatively unscathed—and rehabilitation wouldn't even be considered.

Well, folks, that is exactly what happened. The judge waved the mother's letter before the court and asked the young man,

"Do you know that a lot of people care a great deal about you?" Nod, yes. Then she leveled a fine and probation, and the case was closed.

There was also a legal technicality: it seems that more serious charges (and potentially more DUIs!) would have to come before the court before the judge could mandate treatment for substance abuse in that state. In other words, things would have to get worse before anything legal could be enforced.

No SCRAM ankle bracelet, no rehab in the offing. The mother's words had been acknowledged, and that was all that could happen. She was heartsick. She didn't want the worst for her son; she wanted him to know what he needed to know, that alcohol was ruining his present and could cost him his future. But he had slid through court system one more time. Either he would have to change or the system would eventually get him. Or else.

NONE OF US MADE JUNK

I cite these examples for one reason only. The intervention made in court by an unknown mother for her unknown son was no less heartfelt and worthy than the letters and testimonials made for the son of a Hollywood icon by his father and family and friends—and neither is yours!

Parents, we all know who our children are. Whether we made them from our own bodies or chose them to be our own, we were the ones who guided them into the world. We were dazzled by their sheer perfection, cradled our dreams for them as fervently as we took good care of their growing bodies, reveled in the fun of little-girl- and little-boyhood, and guided them into adolescence with all the wit and wisdom we could muster. Then, through events real and never imagined, some unknown and certainly unforeseen, our children veered into addiction, and we found ourselves living in a different world, with our children as strangers.

As you stumble to your feet in this strange realm, don't give anyone license to dim the light of love you hold for the individual you raised. Detach from your offspring's behavior as you must in whatever way works for you, but do not allow anyone or any system—religious, legal, educational, political, social, professional, you-name-it—to cloud the purity of the love you gave to your child. Cherish your true heart. Honor the purity of your intent. Each will lift your heart when hope weakens and gives way to despair.

You were good then and you are good now. *Protect who you are!* Addiction and its consequences were never what you had in mind, let alone enabling and prolonging it. You only wanted to make life better for your daughter/son. Now the issue is to make YOU better.

LIGHTEN UP

I fully believe that anyone who has been reading these words has done the best that he or she knew how to do at any given time with the circumstances that brought them to their knees. Cut yourself some slack. Lighten up when you need to; make that your new habit. Whether a parent in your position could have cleaned up the mess you are in before things got as bad as they are, remember this: your child made the mess, not you.

Don't beat yourself up over what was never in your control. Take care of your precious self by honoring your powerlessness over addiction.

BIRDS OF A FEATHER

There is nothing noble about going it alone. There is safety in numbers—and solace and inspiration and recognition. Invest your time and spirit with those who understand you. Pooling collective energies will fill in your gaps and theirs; someone else will always have momentum when you don't. They will respect where you are and share what worked for them, or what didn't work when they were in your position. This is no sign of weakness but a mark of intelligence, wisdom, savvy, and strength. You might even help someone else by sharing your experiences.

It's OKAY to need help and lean on others. You would do the same for them. This, Dear Heart, is the genius of recovery groups!

AND BACK TO YOU . . .

In the final analysis, IT IS ALL ABOUT YOU, EXCEPT WHEN IT IS NOT ABOUT YOU. Recover who you are and you will fully inhabit the new world you have entered. Your daughter/son will begin to see you differently and pick up this wake-up signal from you: OOPS, the old rules don't work anymore. The game is over. I need a new gig.

The only "gig" that will heal an addict is to own responsibility for his or her actions, to apply their own strength and awkwardness to the consequences they have earned, and to seize their own power to make better choices about how they are going to live. None of this can happen if they are looking for your reaction to their drama—and your solutions for them.

Be done with drama—theirs first, then yours. You will all calm down, and the air will begin to clear. This is your only way out of the woods into a fresh landscape. Your life has changed forever, but you can become braver, stronger, and wiser than you've ever been. And so can your child.

WILL I EVER GET MY CHILD BACK?

The good news is YES. Recovery is not only possible, but likely if everyone works on him- or herself—that is, recovery from codependence and recovery from addiction.

Living with an addict in recovery is a lifelong process, and presents an ever-fresh array of challenges. The principles of looking after one's self remain the same, and are grounded in one simple premise: *mind your own business.*

Now for the bad news. NO, your daughter/son will never snap back into the dear one you knew before addiction raised its ugly head. Your loved one is changed forever by the spiritual, emotional, and physical assault of substance abuse. And you, Dear Heart, have been changed forever as well by the damaging coping behaviors that have, in fact, turned around to bite you.

There is an expression in recovery: "We never graduate from the program." True statement. Your healing will be lifelong, just as your loved one must make a choice every minute of every day to remain clean. You will have to manage your attitudes, assumptions, and compulsion to fix and manage and rescue and smooth over bumps in the road. If everyone does the work and keeps on doing it, everyone can make it, step-by-step-by-step, one day at a time.

Just keep on keepin' on, Dear Heart, and godspeed.

LIVING THE POWER OF *YES*

YES is the most beautiful word in the English language. My husband and I once put it on a license plate. So my parting gift to you is these words that originated with a very young poet who went by the name of Huckleberry Tao.

One day I'll chase the errant dream
to the edge of aspiration,
Where together we will mount the sky
and ride the wind of Yes.

Take these words as a mantra. They are yours now, from me, from a young woman who was overwhelmed by odds but somehow remained undaunted.

Step forward. Heal. Be well. Be happy. Take off. Take flight.

Know, Dear Heart, that Your Higher Power loves you every day and every night, beyond all days and nights.

• APPENDIX I •

Notes from the Field

Voices of real parents (with un-real names)

who are walking Planet Paradox

JIM AND JEANNE

The expression "It's not the years but the miles" certainly applies to Jeanne, now seventy-three, and Jim, seventy-four. Married for forty-seven years, this congenial pair does not look their age, but they have certainly racked up miles with their addicted son.

Early in their marriage, Jeanne suffered two miscarriages, and the couple adopted a beautiful baby boy, then six months old. Jeanne recalls being told by the adoption agency that baby Matt's birth father "liked to party." A year later Jeanne gave birth to Chad, now forty-four.

Jim and Jeanne were both teachers, and raised their boys in a nurturing home.

Jim notes that his oldest son suffered with frequent respiratory conditions as a child. "Matt would catch a cold and it would go right into his chest, then into bronchitis," he explains. "He could get medication that contained addictive substances for a cough. I can't help but wonder if that made him susceptible to addiction . . ." he says, his voice trailing off. Chad has never abused substances, and does not drink alcohol today.

When Matt was eleven or twelve years old, Jeanne recalls a social occasion for which Jim fixed cocktails. Before their last guests left, they found their son throwing up violently.

"We were stunned that Matt could drink enough to get so sick, so fast," Jeanne states. Jim recalls another occasion when Matt was thirteen, and he drank a six-pack as fast as he could behind the school. By the time he was in high school, they knew his drinking was serious.

"He was always strong-willed and rebellious," Jim recalls. In his senior year, Matt ran a warning light with three passengers in the car, causing a serious accident, and one boy was gravely injured. Jim and Jeanne were sued for one million dollars and were lucky to keep their car insurance after the case was settled, while Matt's insurance was dropped.

"Talk about stress!" Jim exclaims. "He could see what it was doing to us, but was oblivious. He had the most bizarre things happen to him. He was lucky to graduate from high school."

Another incident happened right around Matt's graduation. The family had enjoyed a "relatively calm" weekend at their lake house, joined by Matt and his girlfriend. They left in separate cars at the end of the weekend, but Matt never arrived at home. Subsequently, Jim and Jeanne received a call from a neighbor at the lake who said there was a lot of commotion at their house. Matt and his girlfriend had doubled back, and a big party was under way. Jim called the police and told them to arrest everyone, including his son.

Matt's drinking moved from beer to hard liquor and illegal drugs, and eventually prescription drugs that he abused. As his addiction progressed, he stole from his parents—money, then household items.

Jeanne recalls a silver-plated compote dish of great sentimental value that had been given to them as a wedding gift. One day it disappeared, and she asked Matt about it.

"Mom," he drawled, "it wasn't even sterling silver. I didn't get much for it."

Jim remembers hurricane shutters disappearing from the garage in their Florida home.

"He sold them for the aluminum," Jim exclaims, shaking his head. When he asked Matt about them, he replied, "But you have insurance, don't you? They'll pay for it."

Through the years, Matt was in and out of multiple rehab programs.

"Oh, God, yes," Jim exclaims. "There were so many of them." Two programs he and Jeanne paid for, and for a third their insurance picked up 80 percent. Matt was in and out of halfway houses, a rehab program through a monastery, and programs run by the Salvation Army.

"At each of the places he had so many chances," Jeanne says, "so many people who tried to help him."

At a program in New England, Matt made a friend who took him in after they both got out. Hugh, the friend, stayed in recovery, but Matt couldn't sustain recovery for long. For years he would ricochet between Hugh's house in New England and his parents' home in Florida.

"We'd send him up there on a one-way ticket, and eventually he would end up back on our doorstep," Jim says. "He went back and forth for years."

Jeanne would try to talk and reason with their son. "It was pointless," she said.

"I went off to bed frustrated," Jim says flatly. "Eventually I would break, and the screaming would begin." One night, Jim turned deathly white during a shouting match, and Jeanne became alarmed. Because he had a heart condition, she was afraid he would have a heart attack or stroke. A voice inside her said, "We've got to go." That was in 2003.

The next morning they called a real estate agent in the Blue Ridge Mountains, drove there, and found a house that they wanted to buy. They returned to Florida, sold their home within a week for the asking price, packed up their household, and left without a word to their thirty-eight-year-old son. They had no contact with Matt for two years, and then began writing to him through a friend, who would deliver letters back and forth. The letters were loving at first, Jeanne says, then angry.

Matt's health deteriorated as he got older, and he was put on disability. He took meds for bipolar disorder, ADHD, and multiple ailments, and the accumulation began taking a toll. He was close to death several years ago, and Hugh advised Jim and Jeanne to see their son while they could. They arrived at his bedside in time to watch him rally.

In the fall of 2010, they received another call from Hugh when Matt's condition was again becoming grave. Suffering from full-blown diabetes by then, he was ricocheting among prescription drugs and painkillers. And he was still drinking.

Through a convergence of circumstances that Jim calls a "God wink," they shared a few poignant days together. Two weeks later Matt was dead.

"The only time I respected him was the last time I saw him," Jim says. "I saw the shit he put himself through and tried to turn around."

Jeanne recalls him saying, "I always thought I could go on drinking, and I could be sober."

Their advice to other parents walking in their shoes is straightforward.

"RUN!" Jim says wryly, and then adds, "Get help for yourself as soon as you can." After twenty-seven years, he and Jeanne still attend Al-Anon meetings regularly. "Go only when you're ready," he advises.

Jeanne's advice is: "Early on, let them suffer the consequences, before things get so terrible. All you can do is prolong it."

Their surviving son, Chad, is now forty-four. He is not an addict.

ALEX

Alex is trim and outdoorsy, with dark shoulder-length hair and warm brown eyes. She is newly married and has her hands full. Three out of four children in her newly blended family are in various stages of recovery from multiple addictions. Addiction and mental illness also run on both sides of the family.

Her uncle was alcoholic, and her sister is schizophrenic and bipolar. Alcoholism is rampant in her children's father's family—though he did not drink—and there is "lots of depression," she says. They were married ten years.

Her son, Seth, and daughter, Kelly, were in their early teens when addictive behavior began to surface.

"I thought it was a kid thing," Alex says, "that they wouldn't do it later. We just went on."

Alex took both her children to family counseling that lasted three years, starting around the age of twelve.

When Kelly was thirteen, Alex remembers her getting drunk one night. Her daughter had also begun cutting herself. When Kelly was fourteen or fifteen, she overdosed on Tylenol and had to have her stomach pumped. Two weeks in rehab followed.

"She loved it," Alex says.

After counseling and rehab, things began to even out. Kelly was a good student in high school and went on to college, where she did well—until it came to exams.

"She got good grades 'til finals, then she would binge," Alex says. "I blamed it on the sorority."

She began missing a lot of class, "sick" three or four days at a time. "She was doing Benadryl, and slept all the time," Alex says. "When she was twenty-two, a professor told her that she might as well quit college."

She did drop out, and began working at a hospital until she was fired from that job. "She was getting drunk at lunchtime," Alex says. Kelly was fired from a series other of jobs before she confessed to her mother that she had "a drug problem."

Alex got her daughter into a rehab program, but it did not work out, and afterwards Kelly moved in with a girlfriend nearby. Then there was an incident with a boyfriend.

"She got drunk and took Xanax," Alex explains. "She had her stomach pumped and spent twenty-two hours in the hospital."

Alex brought her daughter home until she could get her into another rehab program for drugs and alcohol in a nearby state.

"It was tough," Alex remembers. Kelly spent five months there.

"Right before her one year of sobriety she relapsed with two drinks," Alex notes. "After that she began AA meetings."

She remembers her son, Seth, as a "great little boy." When he was nine, he began lying and became angry and defiant. Alex, who was a single mother by then, put him in an Outward-Bound-type therapeutic program when he was twelve. The program was residential and lasted thirteen months.

After the ninth grade, Seth dropped out of high school. He earned his GED, and he received a scholarship to college, but Alex insisted that he help pay his way. He refused to work or go to college part-time, so he didn't go at all.

"I couldn't make him do anything," Alex says. "He never finished anything, and couldn't hold a job for more than a few weeks.

"He was irresponsible, but I kept being there for him," she adds.

By age seventeen, Seth was no longer living at home. He married at eighteen and had a little boy. That marriage would end in divorce.

Seth was in and out of his mother's life—living with her, helping in the family business for a while, then stealing checks from her or cash from the business, and leaving.

He would hold a job for a while, then get hurt and start taking pain meds. He was drinking, too, and he would lose his job. He'd move back home, until Alex would make him leave again.

A cycle of getting hurt on the job or in rehab and taking meds and leaving the job or rehab went on for several years. At the age of twenty-seven, Seth finally admitted to his mother that he had been "addicted for a long time."

Alex says her children's father thought she had spoiled both Kelly and Seth as children, and blamed her for their problems. He never paid for any of their rehab or counseling.

Today, Kelly, twenty-five, is in recovery. She is married and working and is the mother of a little boy who is a toddler.

After five months in two different rehab programs, Seth, twenty-seven, is working his own recovery, holding down a job and living on his own. Along the way he had to give up custody of his eight-year-old son.

Alex has been married to James now for less than a year. James helps Alex with the family business. His oldest daughter is a recovering addict, and his youngest daughter is living with them until she graduates from high school. The relationships between and among the blended family members are strained at times, but they are working through it.

Al-Anon has been a huge resource for Alex. She began attending more than two years ago when Seth was moving in and out of her house and the going was rough. She also takes care of herself with exercise, working outdoors, and her "God box." She writes her concerns and fears on a piece of paper, then puts them in the box for God to handle.

Alex seems more confident about her daughter's progress in recovery than with her son's at this point.

"I don't know how he's doing," she states. "I can't trust what he says." But life is getting better as she develops the habit of being good to Alex.

"I still feel guilty about doing things for myself," she says. "Why? I get so mad at myself!"

Her advice for other parents is: "Don't do for them. Learn to say NO. And stand up for yourself.

"Don't be scared," she adds. "They always have a plan."

REGINA AND GENE

A petite, attractive pair, Regina and Gene have been married for forty-seven years and are the parents of Lisa, forty-two, and Mike, thirty-nine. Beyond their concern for their adult son, they have had to help raise two young grandsons.

Addiction runs in both their families. Gene, seventy, is a recovering addict. His father was an addict, and his grandfather died of cirrhosis of the liver. Regina says her father came from a big family of addicts.

"I was functioning, but I didn't like myself," Gene says.

His consulting business kept him on the road a lot when the children were growing up, and he says his wife may have made up for his absences by spoiling them.

"They had everything they wanted, and didn't have to do anything for it," he says. "Mom was too easy on them."

Regina doesn't disagree with him. She adored her children, and says she didn't have a clue when her son's behavior began to change by the age of fifteen, and neither did Gene.

Mike had a best friend whose mother was an RN, and the boys began raiding her well-stocked medicine cabinet regularly. Eventually, Regina and Gene would learn that the boys were taking as many as twenty pills a night.

"We didn't recognize the symptoms at the time," says Gene. "A neighbor told Regina that Mike was on drugs."

"They were poppin' pills and smokin' pot, LOTS of pot!" Regina says. "I couldn't figure out why he was so popular. He was selling it."

Both Regina and Gene finally "got it" about their son's addiction. They knew he drank, but pills were his demon and he did whatever he had to do to get them.

"He stole from us. He pawned things from the house. He stole from our wallets," Regina says.

Mike went into a rehab program when he was seventeen, when Regina says the police were on to him. With the help of two burly neighbors, she and Gene forcibly removed their son from their house and took him to a rehab facility. After their insurance ran out, he was admitted to a day program for a month. He completed about two months altogether.

Early in the tenth grade Mike dropped out of high school, and later earned a GED. He was married at twenty-one, and began dealing prescription drugs with his wife. She worked for a doctor's office and would write prescriptions for them. They also went "prescription shopping" from one doctor to the next. And they had two little boys.

Regina and Gene helped them out financially, first to buy a house. They helped them buy cars. When Mike got hurt on the job and needed two surgeries, they covered his bills. They paid for rehabs and halfway houses and counseling. They paid for Mike to train as a mechanic. They helped with his children.

"Between the ages of fifteen and thirty, I bet he's cost us a quarter of a million dollars of our money," Gene notes. The prescription drug trafficking landed Mike and his wife in and out of jail and on probation or detention at different times. Regina and Gene kept their grandsons during these cycles. After six years, the young couple divorced.

Four years ago, Mike was working at a good job when he failed to pay his tags, car insurance, and driver's license. He was picked up twice in a month and went to jail. Regina and Gene had legal guardianship of the boys. When Mike got out, Gene leveled with him. "Here's the deal: go to rehab or hit the road."

"He had no choice about the second rehab," Regina adds. "He had no car, no money, and no job. I said to him, 'You straighten up or I'm taking these boys, son.' I think that's what did it. He had to face up to his children." During this stressful time, Regina began attending recovery meetings regularly.

Regina and Gene's daughter, Lisa, has suffered from the anguish her brother's addiction has visited upon the family, and Regina believes that she continues to harbor some ill feelings.

She is married and the mother of two, and has never had any signs of addiction.

Mike moved out of his parents' home a couple of years ago and lives nearby with the boys. They visit about once a week for dinner, and their grandparents remain involved in their lives. Mike has been out of work a couple of times, and Regina and Gene continue to help him financially, but he is determined to raise his sons. He drug-tests his boys, who are twelve and fifteen, and he tells them, "Don't think you can get anything past me!"

Though Gene and Regina took the family to church when their children were growing up, Regina says, "So much could have been avoided if there had been more spirituality brought into the home."

"The spirituality that gets to God," Gene emphasizes. He notes that he and Regina received substantial support from colleagues he worked with as a behavioral consultant for companies. They had access to counselors, support groups, and behavioral skills within an accepting environment.

"We did not have to be secretive about it," he says.

Today, church and twelve-step meetings help keep Gene and Regina grounded. Gene has been attending four or five twelve-step meetings a week for seven and a half years, and has been in recovery that entire time. Regina has been attending two Al-Anon meetings a week for three and a half years.

She still gets nervous about how her son is doing, but says, "I never talk about it (his disease) without clearing up something for myself. After years of sharing, I know that lots of people have had it so much worse."

SEAN

Historically, the West has been fertile territory for escape and reinvention, and that is exactly where Sean's son, Wade, headed when the law began snapping at his heels. With $1,800 in his pocket and a place to live waiting, he and a friend headed across the country to start over. Boy, howdy!

Within three weeks the money was gone, the friend was in jail, and Wade was calling his father for sympathy and, he hoped, a handout.

Addiction is the disease of "no matter where you go, there you are."

Sean shakes his head. He is tall and slim, and his salt-and-pepper beard is the only thing that betrays his age, which is fifty-eight. He grew up in an "alcoholic house," and describes his father as a "functioning" alcoholic. Seventeen years ago he lost his wife to cancer, and since then has been a single parent to his daughter Miriam, thirty-two, and Wade, thirty-four. His little granddaughter, Michelle, is three.

His son's addictive behavior began in high school when he was sixteen. Pot and beer were starters. By the time he was nineteen, after his wife died, Sean knew that his son was a serious user. The family went through grief counseling, but Sean says Wade was not a willing participant. He preferred substances.

Wade really can't say what his son's substance of choice is today. "Whatever is going around at the party," he says wryly. "Pot is number one probably, and beer. Meth is really screwing him up, too. And he gets opiates off the street."

His son has become deft at managing his addiction along with his mental conditions. Like many addicts, he suffers from depression. He is also diagnosed with attention deficit hyperactivity disorder (ADHD).

"He gets a diagnosis so he can get the pills," Sean says. "The pot makes him depressed, so he takes speed to go to work."

During his freshman year of college he was busted for possession of pot, but he was able to graduate with a BA in Communications and Sustainable Development.

"He's totally unsustainable," Wade laughs. But he's serious. He says his son can't hold a job for more than nine months. He was in business for himself as a contractor, but nothing has lasted. "He's been unemployed and in deficit condition for the last two years."

Sean admits to reacting badly to his son's addiction.

"I've been angry, judgmental, critical, accusatory, and unaccepting," he says. "It just feeds the reasons for him to do more of it."

Wade has sought help since he became "nonfunctioning" two years ago—medical doctors, community health services. He went into a state-run detox program and lasted a week, and lasted another week in a three-week rehab. He has received outpatient counseling sporadically, but he didn't take to it. He didn't take to twelve-step programs, either.

Run-ins with the law have accumulated, first with speeding tickets. There were vehicle violations when he didn't pay for his registration and license.

He has had no DUIs because he is very careful about how he consumes alcohol. "Pills are popular," Sean says, "because they can't test for them. He wears his hair short and keeps 'the look.' He chews breath mints. He goes to great pains to look normal while acting abnormally," Sean says with another wry laugh.

At one time Wade owned a house; he and his wife were together for seven years and were married for five. All that is gone.

For two years he has been out of work, and Sean notes that he has been in court every month for the last fifteen months. He ricochets among the homes of friends who put him up and feed him until he migrates to the next place. Sometimes Sean feeds him.

"He went out West with a friend to work, to get away," Sean explains. Ever the caring father, he mailed Wade new copies of his driver's license and birth certificate, so he could get a job. "I don't want him coming back," Sean says evenly. But Wade called the other night, homesick and out of money—Sean's son, across the country, living on the edge—and Sean's heart is on the edge with him.

"The worst aspect," Sean says, "is the gut-wrenching fear and anxiety over what's going to happen each day, and the dissolution of the nuclear family, the divorce, the custody battle over his daughter, all the negative energy."

For fourteen years Sean has been attending six recovery support meetings a week. Physical work helps him keep his head clear as he tries to focus on his own life.

"I've become more intent on taking vacations," he adds. He enjoys sailing and camping, and recently returned from a midwinter sojourn to visit friends in Florida for a few weeks.

Sean feels that his biggest shortcoming as a parent has been taking too much responsibility for his son's choices and "being quick to apply guilt and shame to the situation."

His advice to other parents is focused.

"Abandon all your old thoughts and develop new ways of thinking," he says simply.

He holds substantial praise for support groups.

"I always wanted to go it alone, and never understood group. But there is a magic and benefit of the group dynamics. It is a powerful source of support and motivation to do the right thing."

• APPENDIX II •

Twelve Steps for Parents
of Addicted Daughters and Sons

Parents undergo challenges and constraints with

addicted children, no matter what age they are,

that are peculiar to the role of parents. We are bound

to our children for life. The Twelve Steps below

are written for Mom and Dad, to touch you where you live,

where you struggle, and where you can survive to heal who you are.

As we take care of ourselves, we are most likely to meet

our daughters and sons in recovery as well.

1. I HAVE NO POWER OVER ADDICTION or over another's behavior and choices. Investing my energy in business that is not my own has made my life unmanageable and full of chaos. I am powerless over my child's addiction and must step aside so that he or she may take responsibility for his or her choices and recovery.

Babyhood is over; childhood is done. No longer can I protect, rescue, or manage the life of my child. My offspring has a disease that I did not cause, I cannot cure, and I cannot control. The disease of addiction is beyond the unconditional love that I have always felt for my child.

My attempts to rescue and fix my loved one have made my life unmanageable. In trying to control my child's life and circumstances, my own life has spun out of control. I have allowed myself to be driven by anxiety and fear into days and nights of chaos and despair. I cannot continue to live this way.

I do not hold up the Universe—for my child or anyone else—nor should I try, and there is wisdom in accepting that I don't have the power. My work is to clean up my place in the Universe.

My focus is acceptance and surrender.

2. A power greater than I am can restore me to mental, physical, and spiritual health. As I place my trust in a Higher Power of my understanding, I am restored to sanity and serenity.

I look to a power greater than myself for strength and wisdom to live with the disease of addiction without interfering with my child, and to heal my own life.

I am humble knowing there is a grand design beyond my ability to plan or to orchestrate. I have been arrogant in assuming that I have all the answers for my offspring, that I am in charge, and that I can bring about the change that I know is right for someone else—even the one I have raised.

I trust a Higher Power that is always there when I am overwhelmed, anxious, or frustrated and angry. By trusting that I am not alone, I may maintain my serenity.

Giving up my will to be in charge will shift the dynamics with my offspring, allowing him or her to become responsible.

My focus is faith and hope.

3. I am ready to give up my will to control, and allow my Higher Power to direct and protect me.

I have no more resources to offer my offspring. I have exhausted all answers and remedies to control or direct events in his or her life, and with the help of my Higher Power I release this illusion.

I place my trust in the Higher Power that watches over me, and release my child to the care of his or her Higher Power within the grand design that is beyond my vision to perceive. I may not know why my offspring is walking the path of addiction or why I am walking it with him or her, but I accept what is and trust I will be given the strength for what I need to bear and do.

All is in divine order, because a Higher Power exists. I am right with my Higher Power, no matter what happens, and so is my child.

My focus is trust and commitment.

4. I am committed to making a fearless, thorough inventory of wrongs I have committed.

I examine the times and the ways I have hurt my offspring by failing to understand the disease of addiction, that may have abetted his or her pain, guilt, and alienation, and prolonged what is a legitimate illness. I cannot become honest with my child until I am honest with myself.

I examine my behavior, seeking insight as to when I have been accusatory and judgmental, when I have misjudged and berated, and when I have made unrealistic demands.

I trust in the help of my Higher Power to find the courage to be objective and truthful about my wrongs.

I pledge to be thorough in the work I need to do.

My focus is honesty and courage.

5. I admit my wrongs to myself, to my Higher Power, and finally to a trusted witness.

I call upon my Higher Power for strength to enumerate the amends that I need to make to myself and to my child—in that order.

I list my wrongs in writing.

I ask someone with whom I feel safe—a trusted relative, a friend, or my twelve-step program sponsor—to bear witness to my wrongs as I read them aloud. My confidante may discuss and ask questions as he or she feels is appropriate to help me with full disclosure. My listener may also help me recall the many times my actions were helpful and kind. Through the grace of my trusted listener, I express my full humanity.

I thank my Higher Power for the right person to bear witness to defects of character, as well as my assets and I thank my witness.

My focus is trust and commitment.

6. Having articulated my wrongs to a trusted listener, I release them to the Higher Power of my understanding to be removed.

I have nothing to fear. I am safe being less than perfect and fully who I am in the presence of my Higher Power and my confidante. All that I am is accepted. My faults of commission and omission make me human, and I can have compassion with myself.

Through the grace of a power greater than myself, I am free and at peace. I can now fully support my daughter/son without judgment as we meet as equals on a path of recovery.

My focus is willingness.

7. *I humbly ask my Higher Power to remove the wrongs I have recognized as defects of character.*

I trust that my Higher Power will give me the strength to do what I cannot do alone, and lift from my shoulders the defects of character that I have openly recognized and shared with another person.

By doing the right thing for the right reasons for myself with the help of my Higher Power, I am releasing my child into the grace of his or her own Higher Power. With my Higher Power, I am open to a new way of living. I am not alone, and I know that my daughter/son and I are all right—and we will be all right.

I am unencumbered by the past as I move forward.

My focus is faith.

8. I make a list of those I have wronged, and am willing to make amends to them all.

I acknowledge that I have injured my daughter/son with impossible expectations to realize the gifts that I know he or she possesses, and to fulfill my dreams for him or her.

While I aspired to be a perfect parent, I have damaged my self-esteem, believing I was not a good enough parent to keep my child safe, happy, and secure in the life I envisioned.

If I have judged my offspring's other parent for not seeing things the way I did as addiction progressed, for not perceiving the warning signs for our child as I saw them, for enabling behavior that I could see that he or she could not, I acknowledge being judgmental with overreaching expectations. We did not cause, we cannot cure, and we cannot control our child's addiction.

My focus is forgiveness, willingness to change, and accepting responsibility for my wrongs.

9. I make amends to all those I have harmed, except when to do so would cause further harm to the injured party or to others.

How I make amends is up to me. I may do them verbally or in writing with my child. I may make amends indirectly by changing my behavior. I may do a combination of all three. I accept the consequences of making these disclosures and focus on what is most important: that my behavior will change.

Making amends to my daughter/son for my shortcomings as a parent is requisite for my healing to begin, and allows my child to be honest and objective about his or her own shortcomings.

I need my child to understand that I do not have all the answers for him or her, and I am trying to focus on my own truths.

I make amends to my offspring's father or mother for the ways I have judged him or her as a parent and within our relationship. As parents we have loved our child truly, and have done the best that we could do for him or her at the time. That is good enough for the past. What I can do in the future is to resolve to concentrate on healing my own codependence and self-destructive behaviors.

My focus is restitution and reparation, whether directly or indirectly, and accepting the consequences.

10. Every day I take inventory of my behavior and my character flaws as they affect my behavior toward others, and when I am wrong I promptly admit it.

Awareness and objectivity are my foundation. In all my interactions, especially with my offspring, I ask myself whether I am doing the right things for the right reasons, and whether am I minding my own business.

Whenever I start sliding into perfectionism for myself, for my child, or for another, I recognize this as a character flaw, not a mission, and rein in my attitude before I intrude. I ask myself, "How important is it?" I remind myself, "Easy does it." Then I release my compulsion to control other people and events for what I think should be the most benevolent outcome as I remind myself to "live and let live."

My awareness lets me know when I need to adjust my behavior. The flip side of this knowing is accepting myself for being human.

By monitoring my own behavior, I learn to correct my character flaws as they arise within myself. I strive to discard *shouldas, wouldas, couldas,* and *oughtas* from my thinking and to be more accepting, tolerant, and forgiving. I concentrate on the "now" of living, and free my child do the same.

My focus is to be mindful of my own recovery program and remain aware of thinking patterns that lead me astray.

11. Each day I reserve time for spiritual readings and reflection to set the foundation for my day and to maintain spiritual awareness.

In the morning I set aside time for spiritual readings and reflection to set the tone for my day.

I begin in gratitude for the opportunity to live another day as well as I can with the grace of my Higher Power. I remind myself that I do not hold up the Universe.

In all my interactions, especially with my offspring, I strive for awareness in my actions.

In the evening, I reflect on the course of the day and whether I have maintained spiritual integrity. I acknowledge the ways I have succeeded; where I have fallen short, with my child or another, I weigh how I can modify these character flaws.

At the end of the evening, I release the strengths and weaknesses of the day to the Higher Power of my understanding, and thank the Universe for the blessings that are mine.

My focus is to maintain and improve "God-consciousness" in my life and to strengthen my connection to Spirit in the world.

12. I embrace my spiritual awakening for the miracle that it is, and resolve to reach out to others who are suffering as I have and apply these principles in all my affairs.

As I meet other parents whose children suffer with the disease of addiction, I offer empathy and support.

First, I become a heart with ears. I listen. I avoid giving advice; this is stepping out of my business into someone else's, no matter how tempting it may be to make suggestions or make recommendations.

I extend my own experience as it may be appropriate for the person with whom I am talking. I recommend readings that have become trusted resources and organizations and meetings that have worked for me.

I offer my phone number should the person I am talking with need to talk further or become anxious or afraid. I assure him or her that there is hope beginning with ourselves, that our loved ones are more likely to find their way if we free them to do so.

I assure other parents whom I meet on my path that it took others walking with me to help me along, and it will work for them as well.

My focus is giving back what I have received for a greater good.

• RESOURCES •

Addiction in the Family: Stories of Loss, Hope, and Recovery,
by Beverly Conyers (Center City, MN: Hazelden, 2003).

*At Wit's End: What You Need to Know When a Loved One Is
Diagnosed with Addiction and Mental Illness,* by Jeff Jay and
Jerry Boriskin (Center City, MN: Hazelden, 2007).

Beautiful Boy: A Father's Journey Through His Son's Addiction,
by David Sheff (New York: Houghton Mifflin, 2008).

*Choices & Consequences: What to Do When a Teenager Uses Alcohol/
Drugs,* by Dick Schaefer (Center City, MN: Hazelden, 1987).

Codependent No More, Beyond Codependency, and *12 Steps
for Codependents,* all by Melodie Beatty (Center City, MN:
Hazelden, 1986, 1992; 1989; 1992).

Don't Let Your Kids Kill You—A Guide for Parents of Drug and Alcohol Addicted Children, by Charles Rubin (Petaluma, CA: New Century Publishers, 2008).

Feeling Good: The New Mood Therapy, by David D. Burns (New York: Avon Books, 1999).

Help Your Twenty-Something Get a Life . . . and Get It Now: A Guide for Parents, by Ross Campbell (Nashville, TN: Thomas Nelson, 2007).

Letting Go with Love: Help for Anyone Ever Involved with an Alcoholic/Addict, by Mitzie W. (Xlibris, 2005).

Love First—A Family Guide to Intervention, by Jeff Jay and Debra Jay (Center City, MN: Hazelden, 2000, 2008).

No More Letting Go: The Spirituality of Taking Action Against Alcoholism and Drug Addiction, by Debra Jay (New York: Bantam, Dell, 2006).

Setting Boundaries with Your Adult Children, by Allison Bottke (Eugene, OR: Harvest House, 2008).

The Enabler: When Helping Hurts the Ones You Love,
by Angelyn Miller (Tucson, AZ: Wheatmark, 2008).

Tough Love: How Parents Can Deal with Drug Abuse,
by Pauline Neff (Nashville, TN: Abingdon Press, 1996).

*When Our Grown Kids Disappoint Us: Letting Go of Their
Problems, Loving Them Anyway, and Geting on with Our Lives,*
by Jane Adams (New York: Free Press, 2003).

*When Parents Hurt: Compassionate Strategies When You and Your
Grown Child Don't Get Along,* by Joshua Coleman
(New York: HarperCollins, 2008).

*Willpower's Not Enough: Recovering from Addictions of
Every Kind,* by Arnold M. Washton and Donna Boundy
(New York: HarperCollins, 1989).

TWELVE-STEP LITERATURE

Al-Anon's Twelve Steps and Twelve Traditions, revised edition,
Al-Anon Family Group Headquarters (December 2005).

Courage to Change: One Day at a Time in Al-Anon II,
Al-Anon Family Group Headquarters (September 1992).

Hope for Today, Al-Anon Family Group Headquarters (March, 2007).

How Al-Anon Works for Families & Friends of Alcoholics, Al-Anon Family Group Headquarters (July, 1995).

NA White Booklet, Narcotics Anonymous, Narcotics Anonymous World Services, Inc. (1976, 1983, 1986)

Opening Our Hearts: Transforming Our Losses, Al-Anon Family Group Headquarters (2007).

Paths to Recovery—Al-Anon's Steps, Traditions, and Concepts, Al-Anon Family Group Headquarters (August 1997).

• ACKNOWLEDGMENTS •

To my Al-Anon community, oh, my: You have each lifted a light, taken me by the hand, and kept me upright and breathing as we walked, laughed, cried, and kept moving together. Bless. To my sponsor, who allows me to call any time of the day or night and always returns my calls. Bless.

To my writing community: Rogena Walden, thank you for spiritual counsel, editing, proofing, dreaming, and inspiring for more than twenty-five years; Louise Eaton, for your editor's eye, teacher's heart, and love of the written word; Puff Anderson, for original thinking and input; Tom Powell, for skills of inquiry into publishers and for support to persevere. Bless.

To attorney Susan Streible for legal insight. To the late Steve Keenan, a gifted substance abuse counselor. Bless.

To René Colvin for spiritual counsel; to Dotty Ann Malone for insight and constancy; to Qele Smith for heart and spirit and perspective. To Nancy Beery and to Ann Doman for unfathomable compassion. Bless.

To Central Recovery Press, for seeing the wisdom in providing another resource for parents who are overwhelmed and lost in the ravages of addiction in their families. And to my editor, Helen O'Reilly, for her vigilance and heart. Bless.